KICKING UP DIRT

KICKING
UP DIRT

A TRUE STORY OF DETERMINATION, DEAFNESS, AND DARING

Ashley Fiolek

with Caroline Ryder

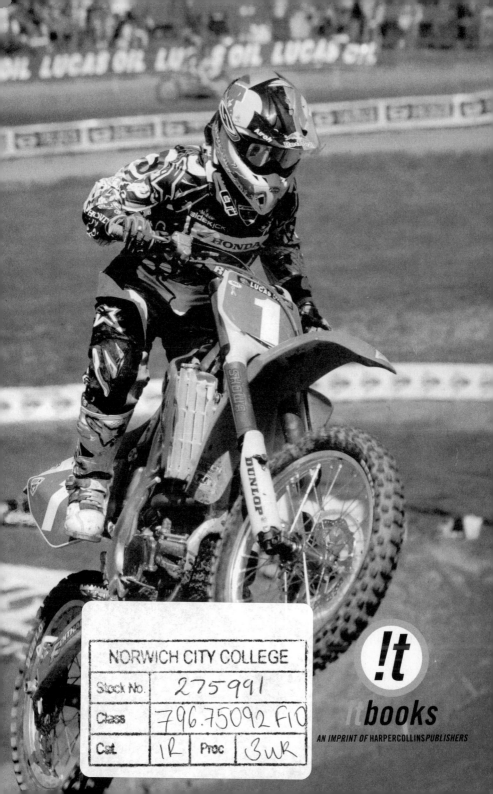

!t
itbooks
AN IMPRINT OF HARPERCOLLINSPUBLISHERS

KICKING UP DIRT. Copyright © 2010 by Ashley Fiolek. All rights re-served. Printed in the United States of America. No part of this book may be used or reproduced in any manner whatsoever without written permission except in the case of brief quotations embodied in critical articles and reviews. For information address HarperCollins Publishers, 10 East 53rd Street, New York, NY 10022.

HarperCollins books may be purchased for educational, business, or sales promotional use. For information please write: Special Markets Department, HarperCollins Publishers, 10 East 53rd Street, New York, NY 10022.

FIRST EDITION

Designed by Ashley Halsey

Library of Congress Cataloging-in-Publication Data has been ap-plied for.

ISBN 978-0-06-194647-9

10 11 12 13 14   OV/WC   10 9 8 7 6 5 4 3 2 1

For Dennis Fiolek, who loved the outdoors, and loved to ride. And for anyone who has a dream and is told it is impossible—nothing is impossible!

CONTENTS

INTRODUCTION: STEEL CITY

The crash happened at Steel City in Delmont, Pennsylvania, during the very last race of the 2009 motocross season. I was only eighteen years old, but people said I was faster on a dirt bike than any other girl in America. All I needed was to finish in eleventh place or higher, and the championship would be mine. I certainly never imagined that I'd end up in the hospital.

At the track, I went through my usual pre-race routine—I prayed with my mom and dad, asking God to keep me safe out there and help me win. Our whole family had worked so hard to get me to this point. We'd lived in motor homes for much of the last decade, chasing the race and chasing my dream. Now *everything* hinged on today. We needed God on our side.

I talked to my mechanic Cody Wolf—we call him C-Wolf—who had arrived at the track the day before to work on my bike. Before each race he strips it apart, breaking it down piece by piece and putting it back together again, so it is born anew.

C-Wolf gave me a broad smile and thumbs-up, indicating that the bike was in perfect racing condition. I felt calmer. At twenty-one, C-Wolf was only a few years older than me, but I trusted him 100 percent.

I went into the motor home to get dressed—knee pads, socks, big racing boots that made me look like I was about to take a walk on the moon. I put everything on in a very specific sequence; it's something I've always been superstitious about. There's so little you can be sure of once you're out on the track—knowing I have put my socks on in the right order gives me one thing to hold on to.

C-Wolf hopped on the back of my red Honda dirt bike—all modern Hondas are red—and we drove through the pit area together, out into the crowd and over to the starting gate at the bottom of the valley. Twenty or so of the nation's top professional racers were lined up to the left and to the right of me, preparing to do battle on the track. I gazed at the rocky Pennsylvania dirt that lay ahead of me. If this track could talk, it'd have some tales—of championship battles, impossible victories, and broken motocross dreams.

The gate dropped, and adrenaline surged through my body. I pulled back the throttle of my 250 cc Honda and it roared into action, propelling me onto the track. After a shaky start, I pushed my way up front. I was in second place, cruising the laps, riding smart and riding steady. The sunshine felt warm on my back as I imagined myself crossing the finish line, and for a second, the championship felt like it might have already been mine.

It came out of nowhere—an unexpected rut in the track. I hit it at an awkward angle and lost control. The bike jolted out from under me and my five-foot-one body slammed to the ground. I felt muscle tearing across my shoulders, followed by a familiar numbness, the sensation of something horribly out of place—*something was broken.* Later, I'd learn that my collarbone had snapped clean in two.

Maybe I should have waited for a stretcher. Maybe I should have let them carry me off the dirt and to a hospital—but I knew if I didn't get back on my bike and finish that race, my championship dreams were over. I heaved myself up, ran over to my bike, and used every remaining ounce of my energy to haul its two-hundred-and-fifteen-pound weight out of the dirt. The handlebars were completely mangled, but luckily the engine was still running. I got on and twisted the throttle, ignoring the pain that accompanied every turn of my shoulders. Dirt spewed out behind my back wheel as I headed in for another lap. The championship wasn't going to wait for me just because I was injured. I was back in the race.

I was wobbly, riding like a grandma compared to how I usually ride. A few of the other girls pushed ahead of me, and I prayed to God, asking Him to help me remain in the top eleven. Behind me, a rookie racer was putting pressure on my position, but I held on tight. I even made a couple jumps to make sure I stayed ahead. By this point, I'd forgotten about the pain—all I could feel was the determination to win. When I crossed the finish line, it was in seventh place—the happiest seventh place I've ever gotten. Even in seventh, I still had the points I needed. *I was the women's motocross champion of 2009.* I felt really glad I had put my socks on in the right order that morning.

Four days later, I was lying in a bed in St. Vincent's hospital in Jacksonville, Florida. I had a hot date with the surgeons, who would insert a plate and six screws into my body the next day. Grandpa Motorcycle—that's my grandfather's nickname—stopped by the hospital to wish me luck. "They puttin' Humpty Dumpty together again?" he said, teasing me. It wasn't the first time he'd visited me in the hospital. Pain, broken bones, and drama—they're par for the course in motocross, one of the most dangerous and least understood sports in the world. It's not traditionally known as a women's sport, and my fascination with motocross is all the more unusual given that I'm profoundly deaf—I've never even heard the sound of my dirt bike. Imagine wearing a soundproof helmet—one that you can't take off—and that's pretty much my world. I've always been at peace with my deafness, though it has definitely gotten me a lot of attention in motocross. Some people can't imagine what it must be like not being able to hear riders coming up behind you—but I've never known any different. Being deaf is fine by me, and it's never stopped me from riding aggressively, like the boys. That's why the inequality in my sport has always frustrated me. In America, men get paid more, they get more practice time on the track, they get the sponsorships, the press conferences, the TV time. But things are changing every year. Women's motocross is evolving like never before, and opportunities that were unimaginable for girls ten years ago are a reality today.

It feels good thinking maybe I had something to do with that—in fact, it makes every broken bone worth it.

KICKING
UP DIRT

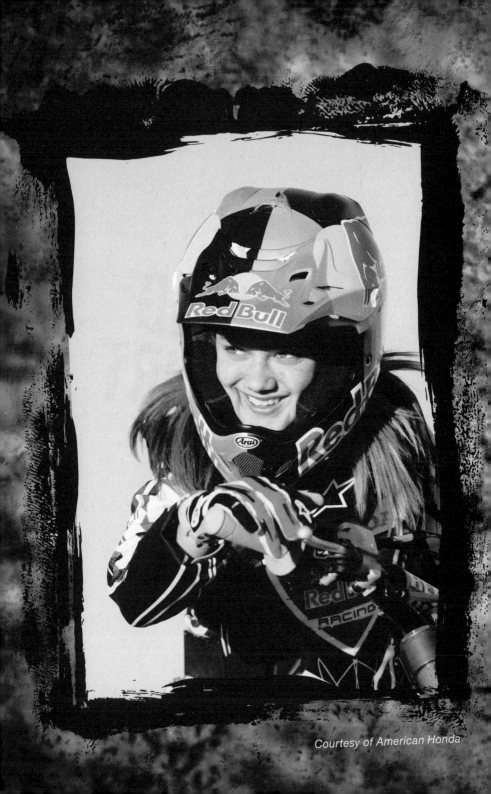

Courtesy of American Honda

FIRST REVS

I was born in 1990 in the shadow of Detroit, in the pleasantly nondescript suburb of Dearborn Heights, Michigan. The Gulf War was brewing, Nelson Mandela had just been released from prison, and Nirvana was about to make it big. I've never actually heard Nirvana—or any music for that matter—but my folks have told me they're very good.

Picture cookie-cutter streets lined with evergreens, oaks, and maples; neighbors chit-chatting over garden fences; Wendy's fast food restaurants and early morning school traffic—my neighborhood was the epitome of suburban normalcy, just one hour's drive southeast of the city.

America's greatest car maker, Henry Ford, was born in the vicinity, and to this day, most everyone in my hometown has gasoline running through their veins. GM, Chrysler, and Ford are headquartered nearby, and on the weekend, rather than going to the zoo, families will go to the Henry Ford Museum and stroll around a replica of the factory where Ford built his first automobiles or take a test ride in a restored Model T. Combustion, ignition, and fuel—those were the things that kept Dearborn's motor running.

My Father, the Dirt Bike Rider

I owe my success to my parents—to my father for believing that little girls can ride motorcycles just as well as the boys, and to my mother for the support that turned my adrenaline-filled dreams into reality. Like all motocross families, they have given up so much—financially and emotionally—so that I could live this life.

Dirt bikes run in my family—my dad, Jim Fiolek, was a motocross racer, as was his father, whose name is Jim Martin Fiolek but whom we call Grandpa Motorcycle. My dad was raised in Dearborn, Michigan, which is circled by Dearborn Heights. He was around five when Grandpa Motorcycle bought him his first dirt bike. At first he wasn't especially interested in it—he was more into hockey. Then when he was around twelve or thirteen he competed in his first amateur motocross race and fell in love with the sport. He always plays down his talent when we talk about his time as a racer. He'll say things like "I was a decent B rider" or "I was just an intermediate." Truth is, I would never be where I am today without the knowledge and skills he passed on to me.

He was racing in the late 1970s and 1980s, a few years after the motocross boom of 1970. Motocross was a simpler pursuit back then—riders would get in their vans and go to the races on the weekend. Now everyone in motocross has a motor home, and the races can last a week. It wasn't an underground sport

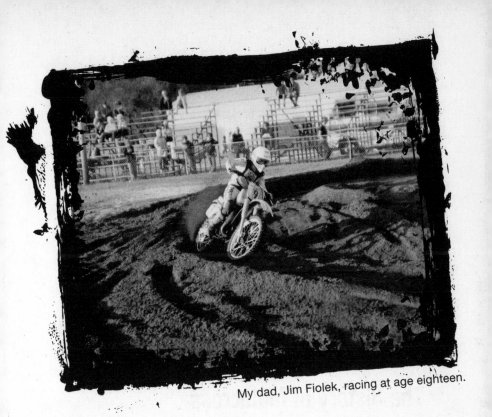

My dad, Jim Fiolek, racing at age eighteen.

by any means—a healthy thousand people or so might have attended a regular weekend race—but the competition wasn't so intense in those days, particularly not among young kids.

The biggest difference between then and now is that the bikes were nowhere near as powerful or as resilient as bikes are today. Modern dirt bikes have incredibly deep suspension—springs and shock absorbers that protect riders from feeling every bump and dip in the track. But back then, there was no such cushioning. With spluttery engines, saddles as comfortable as a wood bench, and a tendency to spit riders into the atmosphere without warning, old bikes had the handling and reliability of a rusty lawn mower. As for *jumping*—only the bravest riders would dare.

Motocross was still recognized as one of the most dangerous sports out there, just as it is today. My dad had his fair share of crashes, as is customary—he broke his ankle, damaged his kidneys, got some stitches. In 1983, after six years of bumps, breaks, and bruises, he decided to quit while he was ahead. He was eighteen and knew he wasn't going to turn pro. With the high risk of injury, he figured there wasn't much point in carrying on unless he was going to take it to the next level. "I reached a point where I started worrying too much about ending up in a wheelchair," he told me. "I knew it was time for me to get a job."

He said good-bye to motocross—for a little while. Once the sport's under your skin, it's pretty much there for life.

The History of Motocross

I tend to live in the moment—but it is important to know the roots of your favorite sport. Motocross is thought to have originated in France (one of my favorite countries). In fact, it was the French who first started calling it "moto-cross." In 1924, the first competition, or "scramble," was held in Great Britain, where the sport was flourishing. In scrambles riders would race their rickety motorized bicycles over roads and natural terrain, traversing foggy marshes and forest streams. "Scrambles" don't have anything to do with eggs—that was the term the Brits liked to use to describe what Americans now call motocross races.

America was watching, and in the same year, 1924, the American Motorcycle Association was born. But only a handful of races took place each year and the sport almost disappeared during the lean years of the Great Depression. Europe would continue to dominate the sport until the very tail end of the 1960s, when a rider called Gary Bailey from South Gate, just outside of Los Angeles, became the very first American to be crowned world champion. His success sparked a homegrown motocross explosion, and the number of races grew a hundredfold in the 1970s, the boom era of American motocross.

In 1972, America birthed its own version of the sport—supercross. The first supercross race took place at the Los Angeles Coliseum at an event organized by rock promoter Mike Goodwin, a motocross enthusiast who was fed up of having to trek around in the heat and dust to watch races. He wanted to create an easier experience for the fans, and that he did. Supercross, housed in stadiums and far easier to televise than motocross, was an immediate hit.

America continued to dominate the global motocross scene throughout the 1980s. In 1987, when President Reagan invited the American motocross team to the White House, it was clear— America had officially adopted the sport as its own. Today, the sport continues to expand and evolve, and is tougher, meaner, and faster than ever before.

Girl Meets Boy

My mom, Roni, was born into a Polish family in Garden City, Lower Michigan, not far from where my dad grew up. Her mother stayed at home and raised the kids, and her dad worked for Ford.

Her parents would never have let her do the kind of wild stuff she lets me do—they were protective of their brood, and my mom and her two siblings led quiet lives growing up.

My mom's parents happened to know my dad's parents, so Roni and Jim grew up aware of one another—vague acquaintances, you could say. But Roni never paid that much attention to Jim until after high school, when they ended up getting jobs at the same place—EDS, a computer company, where they were training to become computer programmers. Roni was nineteen, and Jim was two years older than her. Jim had a serious girlfriend at the time, and my mom was dating here and there. This was around 1987 or 1988.

My dad was always an outgoing, popular guy, and he was known for his obsession with motocross. Physically, he's compact—five foot five and around 120 pounds—but athletic, with steely gray eyes, high cheeks, and a strong jaw. His small frame barely contains his boundless energy. My father has always known what he's wanted and gone after it . . . including my mom, Roni. She is just a little shorter than him, around five foot four, but softer in appearance and in personality. Her hair is a wavy brown, her cheeks are dimpled, and her eyes glow a warm hazel. People say she and I share the same smile. Unlike my dad, my mom was always really shy and kept to herself. She would listen politely when my dad talked to her about dirt bikes—she wasn't even sure what motocross was at the time. That would soon change.

It was at the wedding of a work friend that they acknowledged their feelings for one other, and after dating for around six months, my dad decided that Roni was "the one." He took her to one of the tallest restaurants in America, at the top of the Renaissance Center in Detroit. It revolved slowly and had incredible views of the whole city and of the Canadian border. My mom went to the bathroom to fix her hair, and my dad got on one knee. He waited for her to come back, ring in hand, enjoying the view of the skyline as the whole floor slowly revolved. The view came around a second time, and by the third revolution he was starting to feel antsy . . . had his future wife snuck out and ditched him? He sent a waitress into the bathroom to look for her—and there she was, fussing with her 'do. When my mom finally reemerged, she wondered where my dad was—he was kneeling down on the floor and she couldn't even see the top of his head. She thought maybe *he* had ditched *her* because she had taken so long in the bathroom.

Luckily, it all worked out in the end, and they were married

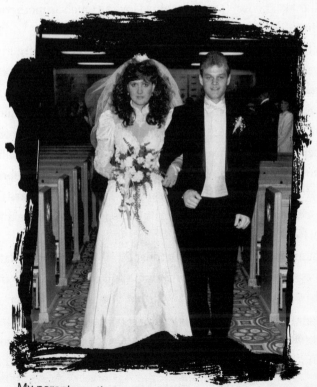

My parents on their wedding day.

in 1989, in a traditional Catholic ceremony in Dearborn Heights. They were young—my mom was twenty-three and my dad was twenty-five—and the first in their group of friends to settle down.

Baby on the Way

My dad has never been one to wait around for anything. When he knows what he wants, he goes for it. First my mom, and then a family. I'm not sure my mom planned on getting pregnant *quite* so fast, but early in 1990, after they'd been married a couple of months, she learned that I was on my way. She started craving ice cream and dairy products while she was pregnant with me, which makes sense—the only thing I love as much as motocross is eating.

While I was in her belly, my mom worked for a contracting company based at the Ford plant. Workers and other personnel were always coming and going—it was a real hub. The doctors who eventually diagnosed my deafness think I might have caught German measles in the womb while my mom was working there. That's the only good explanation anyone has been able to come up with. Normally, deafness is hereditary—but there's no history of deafness in my family, as far as we're aware. In utero exposure to the measles virus is the most plausible explanation for my deafness.

I came into the world on October 22, 1990, two weeks late. My poor mom was in labor with me a full twenty hours—and despite the pain she refused any drugs. She and I are similar in that regard. We'd rather deal with the pain than have any unknown elements injected into our bodies. It's a fear of the unknown. I weighed seven pounds, four ounces, and the doctors said I was healthy and normal as could be. I guess that's how it seemed. In hindsight, there were early signs of my deafness—my mom would be vacuuming under me as I slept in my crib and I wouldn't wake up, for example. It just took a while for everyone to put two and two together.

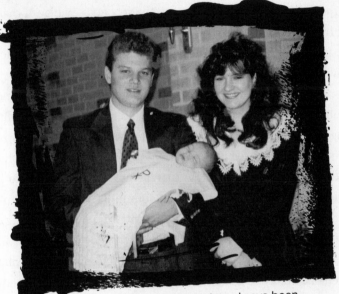

Celebrating my baptism. Faith has always been important to us Fioleks.

"Mildly Retarded"

When I was about one and a half, my mom became concerned that I still hadn't started to talk. My dad had been a late talker, so she assumed that was probably the explanation—but she took me to a pediatrician nonetheless. The doctor examined me and shrugged his shoulders—there didn't *seem* to be anything wrong with me. Just give it time, he said. Six months later, when I still wasn't developing any speech, my mom set up an appointment at the local hospital.

The child specialists there sat me down with some puzzles and tests, simple stuff designed to test intelligence, hand-eye coordination, and so on. Here's the thing—I'm really hyper and sitting still is slow torture for me. Generally I can't even stay put long enough to watch much TV. As you can imagine, I lost interest in the doctors' tests almost the second they placed them in front of me. Based on my decidedly ADD performance, they deduced that my inability to talk was due to mental deficiency. I was "mildly retarded," they said. On top of that, I was "lazy," and my parents should stop "spoiling" me. "If she points at something, don't get it for her," they said. "She should learn to say what she wants." The news sent my parents into a tailspin. *Mildly retarded?* First they felt shock . . . then confusion . . . then anger. It didn't make any sense—other than being silent, I seemed pretty bright to them. If they said "Go get your milk," I would go get my milk. What they didn't realize was that *I was already learning to lip-read.*

In the end, it was my mom, not the doctors, who finally figured out what was going on. One day, she accidentally dropped a bunch of pots and pans behind me, and I didn't flinch. She thought this seemed odd, so she took some more pans up behind me and started banging them, right there. I didn't react. That's when she began suspecting there might be something wrong, not with my intelligence but with my *hearing*. Six months later, specialists at the University of Michigan confirmed her suspicions—I was profoundly deaf. They diagnosed me almost immediately, after a series of tests. The tests took place in a dark room, and I sat on a chair with my parents behind me. The specialists observed how I responded to various noise-making tools—like monkeys with cymbals and other toy animals. Of course, I didn't respond—I couldn't hear a thing. Having endured a year of not knowing what was wrong with me, the news came as a relief to my parents. Finally they knew what the real problem was. And this time it didn't feel like a mistake.

We were ushered into a small office with one of the specialists straightaway. "I am going to teach you a few very basic things," he said. This would be our very first introduction to sign language. He showed us how to sign words like "apple" (made by closing your hand and placing the knuckle of your right index finger against your cheek) and "milk" (made by clenching either hand). My mom says she'd never seen me look so happy—at last, we could communicate with one another!

The doctor asked my parents if they'd consider getting me fitted with cochlear implants, electronic radio devices that are surgically implanted behind the ears, beneath the skin. They can help extremely deaf people like me develop some hearing sensation—but one of their downsides is that any kind of physical impact can be dangerous for the wearer. As such, they limit the amount of contact sports you can participate in. My mom and dad talked to other young deaf people and most of them said the same thing: "Don't get the implants!" For several years, doctors would urge my parents to reconsider implants, but they didn't feel comfortable making a decision on my behalf. When I was around eight years old, in third grade, they discussed it with me seriously. They said they would support whatever decision I made. But I felt the same way they did—I was fine the way God had made me. I'm so grateful they didn't just steam ahead and have the surgery done. My life would have been very different if they had; I might never have become a motocross racer. Even today, we talk about it and I know I'll never get the implants—I don't even want a hearing aid. Not that it would make any difference.

Several members of my family were appalled by the news of my deafness. And it didn't help that my parents seemed so relaxed about the situation. After all, to many hearing people, deafness seems like a tragedy. They can't imagine a world without music, for instance, or going through life without knowing what your name sounds like. Well, I've never known any different. To me, being deaf doesn't feel tragic at all. I just have a different way of experiencing things.

Immediately after the diagnosis, my parents drove me up to Northern Michigan to visit Grandpa Motorcycle. During the drive, they started figuring out a plan of action, laying out some broad goals for themselves and for me. First things first—they were going to learn sign language, so they could communicate with me. Then they would research schools for me. It all seemed surprisingly manageable to them. In fact, people sometimes wonder why my parents *didn't* freak out more when they found out about my deafness. But it's just not their style. My mom and dad have always rolled with the punches and adapted to whatever God has given them. Their reaction, or the way they describe it to me, was, "OK, cool. She's deaf. Now at least we know what we're dealing with." Grandpa Motorcycle was almost as calm as they were about my deafness after the initial shock, at least. The way he saw it, if his son and daughter-in-law were OK with it, then so was he.

It took a few moments for the dust—and the emotions—to settle. Then the whole family started the process of adjusting. There was a whole new world for us to explore.

Total Communication

In my family, we've become very used to having to fight for things, and one of our very first battles was with the state of Michigan. At the time, Michigan was an advocate of "oral deaf education," in which the focus is on learning to speak and lip-read combined with use of hearing aids and cochlear implants, rather than a sign-language-based education. But my parents were more drawn to the alternative, a "total communication" program, which places as much value on signing and finger-spelling as it does on things like lip-reading and voice.

My parents found themselves pressured to put me in an oral program, a path they didn't feel was quite right. In their opinion, American Sign Language offered a more effective way for us to communicate with one another—but the state insisted my parents at least visit an oral program before making a decision. So they did—my mom and dad checked out an oral program nearby and visited four or five different classrooms.

"Every classroom was filled with kids working on saying the word 'apple,'" she later told me. "They seem to spend all day trying to say this one word!" By this point anyway, I was already signing the word "apple." I could also sign what *color* apple I wanted, and how many pieces. My parents felt it was more important that I spend my days following a regular curriculum of math, English, and science, so they stuck to their guns, and we started a home-based total communication program straightaway.

Hearing babies start absorbing language right after they are born—but I was nearly three years old, and I had almost no concept of language whatsoever. We had some catching up to do. My parents enrolled me in a preschool program with hearing kids for a month. A sign language professional started coming over to our home twice a week, working for an hour with my mom and me. The first few sentences we learned were really basic—like "What do you want to eat?" and "Do you have to go to the bathroom?" Then my mom took photos of everyone in the family, and next to each person's photo, I would draw his or her sign name, which was always based on a memorable object or thing I associated with that person. That's how we came up with "Grandpa Motorcycle." Deaf people often create shortened sign language names for their friends and family, based on whatever thing they remind you of the most. My grandma on my mom's side, for example, had a dachshund, so she became "Grandma Hot Dog." I had always associated my dad's dad with motorcycles, so he became "Grandpa Motorcycle." Now that's what everyone calls him.

My mom says I was good at signing right off the bat. Within a year of my diagnosis, I was able to ask for all my favorite foods in sign language. When I was three and a half I enrolled at a school in Dearborn called Whitmore Bolles Elementary, a hearing school that made special provisions for deaf kids. Academic classes were with deaf students, and I could interact with the hearing kids more closely during activities like PE and Girl Scouts. I attended Whitmore Bolles from 1994 to 1998.

In hindsight, I know I was lucky that my parents were willing to invest so much of their time into helping me communicate—so many of the deaf kids I met at school, those born into hearing families, told me their parents hadn't been able to invest much time into learning sign language with them. The Fioleks, on the other hand—we had a whole language of our own going. McDonald's was two little arches with your fingers, for instance. And there were more personal signs—whenever I was acting up or getting hyper, my mom would take the palm of my hand and run her fingers over the edge of it until they fell off the edge. "You're over the edge, Ashley," she would laugh, and immediately I would calm down. Just something about feeling her hand on mine made me relax. In public I was shy, but when at home with my family I could be incredibly boisterous, never wanting to sit down or stay still. "You were an angel child at school, and at home you were a hellion," my mom jokes today.

In the meantime, my mom and dad had started taking adult sign language classes at night school. And they made friends with other deaf families, families that "adopted" us and introduced my parents to the deaf way of life. My folks would be invited to parties where, quite often, they were the only hearing people in the room. My mom admits it was hard to adjust at first. But they were supremely grateful for the love and acceptance of the deaf community, a community my parents had no experience with whatsoever.

My dad was just as involved as my mom when it came to learning sign language and to learning about deaf culture, which was unusual, my parents learned. Apparently, when hearing parents have a deaf child, it's generally the mother who takes on the burden of cultural integration. But my dad was all over it. He had so many things he wanted to talk to his little girl about, after all—like motocross.

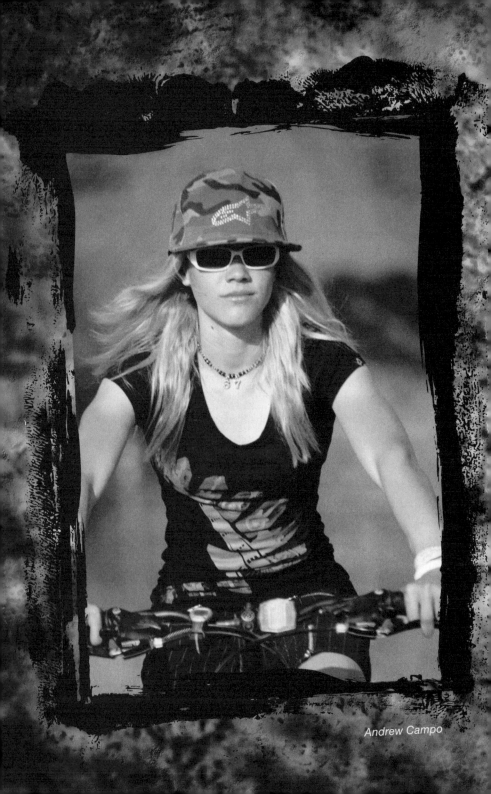

Andrew Campo

chapter 2

THE GATE DROPS

Grandpa Motorcycle

Grandpa Motorcycle, my dad's dad, has had faith in me right from the start. They say he's my number one fan, and he follows me to races all over the country. He hates to fly, so he's logged thousands and thousands of miles in his old Ford truck, criss-crossing the nation in the name of motocross. Like my dad, he's small. Unlike my dad, he has a thing for wild-colored jean shorts.

There's no doubt the Fiolek obsession with dirt bikes started with him. In the 1970s, while living in Dearborn and working at General Motors, he cofounded a road bike club called Kings and Queens. This hobby segued into motocross and enduro racing—trail racing in the woods for long periods of time. In enduro you don't go as fast as you do in regular motocross, but you do have to weave through the woods for hours and hours, navigating

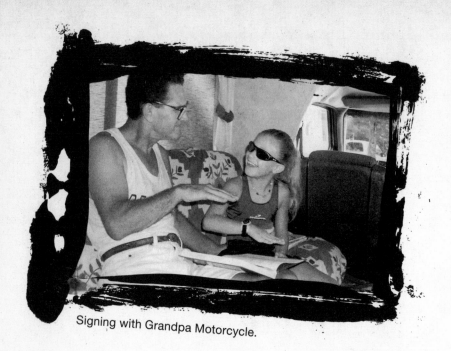
Signing with Grandpa Motorcycle.

gnarled roots and overhanging branches. It's not for the faint of heart.

The first time I ever got to ride a motorcycle was up at Grandpa Motorcycle's cabin in Wolverine, a forest town in Northern Michigan. There isn't much to do—only a couple of restaurants and no movie theater—so you pretty much have to make your own fun.

I was just one and a half years old when my dad sat me on the gas tank of his bike. We disappeared into the woods, following the trails, with mom on her quad next to us. That's my earliest memory—being on the front of my dad's bike, feeling like I never wanted to stop. If they did ever pull over because it started raining, I would start yelling and bawling. I guess the cold and wet never bothered me—they still don't.

You could say we've always been an outdoorsy family. I mean, who wants to watch TV when there's a whole world of fun waiting to be had outside? Even in the winters, which tend to last forever in Michigan, we'd make the three-hour trip up to Wolverine every weekend. We didn't care about the freezing wind and the snow—my dad would hook up snowboards to the back of my mom's four-wheeler, and we'd scoot around for hours in the ice and slush. Going through muddy winter puddles was always so fun—sometimes it was hard to tell just how deep they really were. There's nothing quite like parting the brown waters on your bike and emerging on the other side, soaking wet.

I've been riding in chilly conditions since I was young, and it's helped me deal with extreme weather as a professional motocross racer. With the cold, I get to a point where I just don't feel it anymore. And on the rare occasions that it does bother me, I just think about Grandpa Motorcycle's cabin and how there was

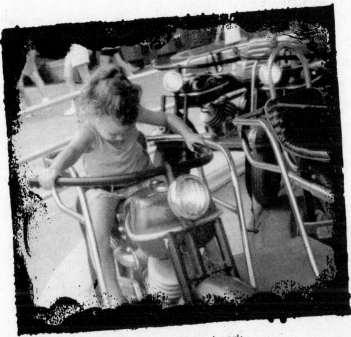

My first solo "ride" at an amusement park.
Faster, please!

always a crackling fire and a cup of hot chocolate waiting for us inside. That always warms me up, even if it's only in my head.

In the summertime, the weather in Michigan flipped to the opposite extreme—we'd spend languid humid days swatting away clouds of tiny bugs and drinking lemonade. But so long as I was moving, I didn't mind the stickiness—the breeze kept us cool. We would see deer, squirrels, and raccoons as we wove through the Wolverine forest, and even in its thickest depths, we never felt alone. The forest, the riding, the pine-scented air— everything about Grandpa Motorcycle's cabin was magical, and even though he sold it a few years ago, it holds a special place in my heart. It always will.

Forest Ranger

The cabin sat at the top of a hill, and at the bottom was a small dirt track with a couple of little jumps. My dad learned to ride on that track when he was a little kid, and that's where he first put me on a bike too, before I could even walk. He had bought me my first bike, a Yamaha PW50, a tiny little thing with training wheels. Perfect for a three-and-a-half-year-old speed freak like me! It cost my parents around $1,000, which was a lot of money for them, but they had a feeling it was something I really wanted. How right they were!

One day, up at the cabin, my dad pointed to the track at the bottom of the hill.

"You want to go down there on your new bike?" he signed. I nodded. It was time for my first real ride.

The track was overgrown, riddled with roots and vegetation, so my mom and dad spent a full day clearing it, getting it ready for my big debut. Because I was so young, only three years old, the memories are foggy, but my parents tell me I zoomed round and round on that little baby motorcycle for hours. When I fell off—which was every few minutes or so—they'd pick me up and put me back on. I'd be whooping with excitement and laughing, according to my mom, who was amazed at my already insatiable appetite for riding.

Soon enough, the little dirt track at the bottom of the hill just wasn't cutting it anymore—I was five years old and ready to hit the big time. I wanted to be riding out in the woods with my parents and Grandpa Motorcycle—not sitting on my dad's lap. I begged my parents to let me go out with them. They didn't need too much convincing; they have always encouraged the daredevil in me. As has Grandpa Motorcycle.

"Let the girl ride her bike," he told my parents. "If she thinks she's ready, she's ready."

They dressed me up in my kids' gear. Little helmet, knee pads—the works. The weather was beautiful—it was spring and the ice had just melted. I still had my training wheels on, and I couldn't wait for the day my dad would unscrew them—but that was still a few years down the line. For now, I was just excited to be going on my first big solo ride among the pine and birch trees that surrounded the cabin.

My dad took off first, on his green Kawasaki. He signaled at me to follow him. I twisted the throttle on my minibike and followed his lead as we headed out into nature. All I've ever known is silence, but somehow the quiet in the conifer woods feels heavier. I caught sight of the shadow of my mother's four-wheeler behind me. I knew she was there, keeping an eye on me. I figured Grandpa Motorcycle was right behind her. Most people, when they're riding, can hear people coming up behind them, and they use their voices to communicate with one another, shouting over the sound of the engines. Because I can't hear anyone or anything, I was already starting to use my sixth sense, my rider's instinct, observing each and every change in my surroundings, always staying alert for any possible obstacles ahead of me.

After a half hour on the trails, we came upon a tarmac roadway. My dad signaled for us to follow him, and we rode single file along the side of the road. We must have looked like quite the little motorcycle family—three generations of Fioleks doing what they love best! I saw a restaurant ahead of us in the distance, and my dad signalled for us to pull into the parking lot. My parents let me walk into the restaurant first, and I strolled in holding my little helmet under my arm, feeling proud as could be.

During those years, between the ages of three and seven, riding was just for fun. None of us thought about my racing. The only knowledge I had of competitive motocross was gleaned from sitting on my dad's lap while he watched motocross championships on TV. In the nineties, motocross wasn't on the television very often—if you did catch a motorcycle race on TV, it would generally be supercross. But on those days when a motocross race was on the tube, it became a family occasion, and we would all sit close together and cheer on our favorite riders. My dad used his basic sign language to tell me tales of epic battles between champions in the mud, and I lapped them up. I wished I knew what it felt like to speed around a track with a bunch of other kids on bikes.

Motocross vs. Supercross

Motocross and supercross are two sides of the same action-sports coin—the major differences lie in the length of the track, and the jumps. Today, jumps are among the most exciting—and daunting—elements of a motocross race, in which a rider speeds up to a dirt hill and is sent flying into the air. A double jump consists of a series of two mounds, and in a triple—one of the toughest jumps to pull off—the rider clears all three mounds in one jump. They are the highlight of any motocross race today.

In motocross, double and triple jumps are high-speed, long-distance maneuvers that require momentum and steady rhythm. In supercross, jumps are more numerous, and they are steeper, almost perpendicular—the kind that will shoot a rider straight up in the air. Technical precision and nerves of steel are required to be a supercross star.

Supercross has a bigger following, partially because the competitions are set up like concerts or baseball games, taking place in metropolitan-area stadiums that can hold fifty thousand or so fans. Supercross is accessible—spectators might visit the stadium to watch a concert one week and then return the next week to watch a supercross race, regardless of whether they have any connection to motorcycles or supercross whatsoever. Motocross, on the other hand, is rural, and races will take place out in the boonies. And its fans generally have some kind of family connection to the sport. Perhaps they raced or their father raced—either way, they tend to be hard-core.

The first real race I ever went to was at an indoor stadium in Detroit called the Pontiac Silverdome. It was a supercross race and I remember munching on hot dogs and popcorn, transfixed by the spectacle going on below us. In 1996, when I was six years old, my parents bought their first motor home—a Coachmen Catalina Class C—and that allowed us to start traveling around the country so I could see the different types of tracks and races. In 1997 we went to the Mini Olympics—a huge amateur race down in Gainesville, Florida—and watched a young James Stewart work his magic on the track. (James is one of today's biggest motocross stars and a hero of mine.) Sitting up there in the bleachers, watching real racing, my perspective shifted. For the first time, I actually saw people riding not just for fun, but to *win*.

"I Wanna Race!"

In 1998, my mom, my dad, and I took a vacation to Florida. We were supposed to hang out at Disney World but ended up spending all our time riding at an ATV park called Croom Forest in Brooksville. That's where I told my dad to take off my training wheels. I was ready to ride—for real. Perhaps I had been inspired by watching the professional races. Or maybe I had grown more confident. Either way, my folks were delighted—they had been encouraging me to get rid of the training wheels for a while, mainly because they actually made riding more difficult for me. The bike would always lean to one side or the other when the wheels were on, making me feel like I was going to fall off.

So off came the training wheels, and off I went. I rode around in a circle for a few minutes, but that wasn't enough. I told my mom and dad I wanted to follow them through the woods while they rode their bikes. They looked at each other, surprised, but they agreed to let me do it. I zoomed around behind them for hours, no training wheels and totally independent. No longer wobbling and out of control, I finally felt at ease on the bike and like it could take me anywhere. It was a whole new feeling. When we got back to the motor home, I knew I had fallen in love with motorcycles. There was no going back.

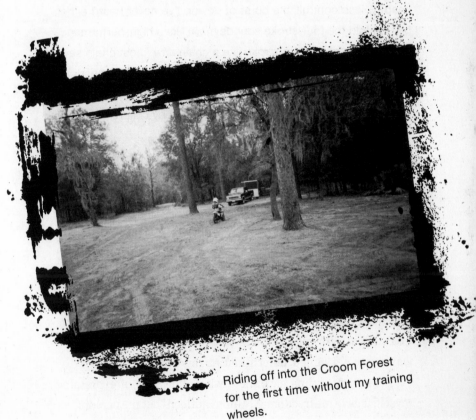

Riding off into the Croom Forest for the first time without my training wheels.

Four-Stroke Versus Two-Stroke Engines

Modern off-road motorcycle racing is done with either a two-stroke engine or a four-stroke engine. The four-stroke delivers a smooth broad range of power, and the two-stroke delivers a snappy, less controllable burst of power. I've never heard either, but I'm told the four-stroke sounds more like a high-performance car engine and the two-stroke like a chain saw (most chain saws have a two-stroke engine). The sport is graduating to nearly all four-stroke motors, with two-strokes still found in the amateur ranks, especially on smaller machines raced by children.

The next day we went to Pax Trax in Bunnell, Florida—a real motocross track. I tore it up on the kids' peewee track, which is shorter, gentler, and less treacherous than an adult track. I must have gone round and round it nonstop for a good three hours. Out of the corner of my eye I could see the big track. Every lap I would stop, look at my dad, and point at it. He would smile and sign, "No, not yet." The big track was for racing, he explained. "Well, I wanna race!" I signed, determination on my muddy face.

Being deaf, riding gave me a whole new way of expressing myself. It gave me freedom. My mom noticed that my personality started changing—before motocross, I was introverted, clinging to my mom and dad whenever I met new people or was in unfamiliar places. But motocross made the outside world less scary. I became eager to get dressed and leave the house, because I knew that being outside meant we might get to go riding. As a rider, I could walk up to a group of motocross kids and feel like I belonged, because we all had one thing in common—we loved the dirt. Motocross was helping me escape the silence in my head and connect with the outside world.

My First Race

Right after coming home from Florida my dad went on the Internet to look for races happening nearby. I had said I wanted to race, and he wasn't going to wait around so I could change my mind. He knew the Michigan amateur circuit pretty well, having worked it himself, and picked a race called the Spring Fling at a track called Log Road in Coldwater, Michigan. Held in March, it's one of the earliest races in the motocross calendar. At that time of the year, Michigan's tracks are generally pretty wet and muddy—but I don't think any of us had any idea just how miserable the conditions would be. My parents almost didn't let me enter when they saw how slippery the track looked, thinking that they didn't want my first experience of racing to be about a mud bath. But I wasn't giving up that easily. All I wanted to do was race—no matter how muddy it was out there. Eventually my parents relented and let me line up with the other kids.

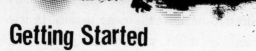

Getting Started

If you've never ridden a dirt bike before, just be warned—once you get on that track, there's often no going back. Motocross is an enormously addicting sport, provided you have the right blend of patience, determination, and daring. A high pain threshold helps, too.

You first step should be to find the right bike—I recommend you start with something that doesn't have too high an engine capacity, and don't forget to learn basic bike maintenance. Try joining motocross message boards to find good deals on used bikes—you'll find some steals at the end of the season or when new models come out and riders want to trade up.

If you're just starting out, buy secondhand gear—there's no point in spending a ton of cash on brand-new gear, especially if you're young and still have some growing to do. You should buy a new helmet, though—that's the most crucial part of any rider's gear. Start getting fit. Motocross is tiring, and you'd be surprised at how many crashes happen just because the rider is exhausted.

Visit sites like mxsports.com, which will guide you in how to get started as an amateur racer. There are important rules and regulations every rider needs to be aware of. Walk the track before you race it, and then, during your practice session, look for all the different lines you can take. Always wash your bike between races—mud is heavy, and can slow you down. Oh—and don't be late to the start line. Early mornings and long drives are part of the motocross lifestyle.

And as you improve your technique, check out the many videos on YouTube in which experienced riders share the secrets of their technique. There weren't too many videos when I first started out, now the internet is packed with amazing information for the beginner motocrosser.

These days, there's no excuse not to become good!

There were twelve of us peewee riders, and while I can barely remember anything of the race itself, I know I did pretty well. I came in fourth and I got to take home a little trophy. I held it tight all the way home. This was my first taste of winning, and I liked it. I think that's when my parents realized that I wasn't kidding around when I said I wanted to race.

Every weekend after that, all I wanted to do was race. My new obsession with dirt biking was unnerving at first for my mom because like all novice motocrossers, I would fall off the bike all the time. But I'd always bounce right back up again. My mom often observed that her friends' kids were always bashing themselves up just playing in a playground or scooting around on their bicycles—yet I'd be on my dirt bike and not get bumped or bruised half as much as they did. I guess I was tougher than I looked.

Of course, it helped that I was well protected—I wore all the gear. Even when you're just starting out, you simply can't ride without full gear. You need it to protect you from the heat of the bike and the impact of falling. Because falling is what motocrossers do best. Bearing that in mind, we dress to protect: our pants are made from thick canvas material with leather patches strategically sewn on where the hot exhaust pipes could possibly burn us. We also wear jerseys, like regular football or sports jerseys, made of thin, breathable fabrics—if it's cold, we can just add layers underneath. Jerseys are always long sleeved in motocross, which helps protect us against the "roost"—the rocks and dirt that shoot up behind riders. Get caught in someone's wake as they go around a corner, and you'll be "roosted"—never a pleasant experience. Of course, we always wear a helmet—with full-face coverage, for maximum protection—and goggles. Our boots are tough too—leather with steel toes and thick soles. I also wear a neck guard, even though it is not required. And I usually wear a chest protector—but not always.

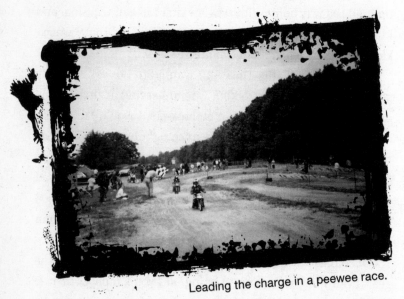

Leading the charge in a peewee race.

My dad would like for me to be even better protected—he is always trying to persuade me to wear a kidney belt to support my innards. There's so much bumping up and down in motocross, it can permanently shake you up on the inside. When he was racing, he didn't wear one and now his kidneys are really weak—he's always racing to the bathroom. The kidney belt, which looks kind of like a tool belt and sits under your jersey, is supposed to hold your internal organs in place so they don't bounce around too much. Most riders don't wear them and I never really liked them because they always felt too big for me. Feeling comfortable is sometimes more important to me than feeling protected.

Feeling the Bike

Soon I moved up from an automatic 50 cc bike to a manual 65 cc bike. That's when I faced my first real challenge on a dirt bike: learning how to shift gears. Most riders know when it's time to change gears by the way the engine sounds—if it's screaming, you shift up; if it's chugging, you shift down. Not being able to hear anything left me at a major disadvantage, one that could have prevented me from ever getting really good at riding a dirt bike.

Thankfully, my parents don't think there should be any limitations placed on me just because I'm deaf. So when it came to shifting, my dad said we simply had to figure out another approach. Some friends suggested we install a red light on my bike that would light up every time I needed to change gears. But having to keep an eye on a light at the same time as watching the track would have been impractical. Instead, my dad devised a different solution—he taught me how to feel my bike.

When the bike was revving he would make a sign. "When you feel it like that, it's time to shift," he signed. It took me a while to get the hang of it—sometimes I'd flip over the handlebars if I accidentally put the bike in neutral at the wrong moment. But we kept on at it. Eventually, my body learned how to tune in to the changing vibrations of the engine. I became so connected with my bike, it became almost like an extension of myself. Today, I always know when things aren't right—because I can feel it.

People often ask me to explain what "feeling the bike" actually feels like. Well, it's like a whole-body kind of thing, with each part of me absorbing information from the engine. The motor sends vibrations through me in every place I am touching it—my legs, my hands, my toes. I don't consciously think about feeling my bike anymore; it's become instinct. And it's something everyone could do if they tried. Maybe they should teach more motocrossers to feel the bike. Because in the long term, I think it's made me a better rider.

Between 1994 and 1998, as well as learning to ride my dirt bike, I was learning what it meant to be a deaf person. It was as though I was exploring two entirely different worlds, both of which would shape my identity in so many ways. When I wasn't riding, I was going to school at Whitmore Bolles, learning sign language and making friends in the deaf community. I was a Girl Scout, which I loved (an interpreter from Whitmore Bolles would go with us), and I started taking gymnastics, ballet, and jazz dance classes in Dearborn. Almost always, I was the only deaf kid in the room.

Then I made a good friend, Britnee Hursin, who was in my class at school. She was hard of hearing, and we immediately bonded. Her brother, mom, and grandmother were all deaf, so she knew how to sign really well. She was the only other child I'd met who I felt could relate to my experience of the world. Britnee was my first best friend, and we did everything together—we went to school together, we took dance classes together, we bugged our parents to take us to McDonald's together. Britnee's mom took it upon herself to show my family the ropes, introducing us to their deaf friends and inviting us to parties.

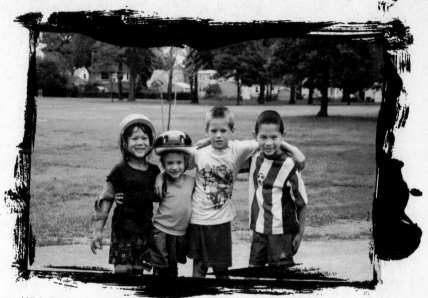

With Britnee (left), and two of our other deaf friends from Whitmore Bolles Elementary School, Jarvis Beaver and Andrew Hursin (Britnee's brother).

When Britnee and her family left Michigan and moved to California in the summer of 1998, it left a hole in our lives. So much so, that my parents started reconsidering whether Michigan was in fact the best place for us. With Britnee and her family—our good friends—gone, coupled with the lack of good schools for deaf kids *and* the state's pushy oral policy—suddenly Michigan didn't feel like a place we wanted to call home anymore. We felt drawn toward a warm climate and started looking at their options. It came down to a choice—California or Florida.

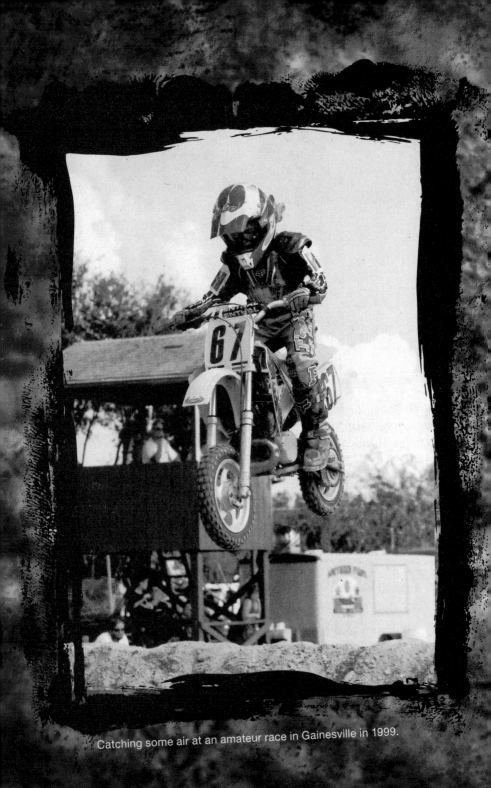

Catching some air at an amateur race in Gainesville in 1999.

chapter 3

FLORIDA DIRT

Sunshine, at Last

In August 1998, my mom, my dad, and I said good-bye to Michigan and headed south, to sunny Florida. Our new home was in St. Augustine, a history-steeped colonial city in the northeastern part of the state, about thirty miles from Jacksonville. St. Augustine was the first settlement established in the U.S. by the Europeans and is the oldest port in America. My mom would find old Indian arrowheads in the land around our house—unsurprising, as several native tribes lived in the area before it was conquered by the conquistadors, led by Juan Ponce de León, the first Spanish explorer to arrive in Florida. Legend has it that Ponce de León arrived in St. Augustine in search of the fabled Fountain of Youth, whose magical waters gave the drinker the gift of agelessness. Today, there's an actual fountain in town, and thousands of tourists flock to it each year, hoping perhaps to erase some laugh lines. The fountain, the history, the people—older folks, deaf people, and a large gay community—give St. Augustine a colorful flavor all its own.

Even though our new house was barely eight miles from the ocean, it felt pretty rural, on ten acres surrounded by sand, sand, and more sand. At night my dad would light fires and invite friends over—he's always been a social guy. The back was secluded enough that my dad could build me a little practice track, and I'd drive my dirt bike on it all day, until the sun went down. After the cold dark winters of Michigan, stepping into this southern dreamland with its perpetual sunshine and turquoise coastline was a little unsettling. I was used to four very different seasons—but in Florida, each long sunny day blends into the next. The climate wasn't the only reason my parents picked St. Augustine—the Florida School for the Deaf and the Blind (FSDB) was the main attraction. It's the biggest school of its kind in America. Ray Charles, the famous blind jazz pianist, is its most famous alum, and it is government funded, so my folks didn't have to pay for me to go there—which helped, of course. Money's always tight when there's a motocross kid in the family.

I joined the school in third grade, one of around eight hundred students. Some were blind, but most were deaf, like me. We followed a regular Florida curriculum of English, reading, writing, math, and science, tailored to fit our needs. Coming from a school and community where I was one of very few deaf people, this exposed me to a whole new world. Suddenly I wasn't in a minority anymore. For me, a kid who came from a hearing family, being immersed in a world where everyone was like me was life-changing.

Even the city itself felt more welcoming—because of the school, there were deaf people *everywhere*. Go to any restaurant in St. Augustine, and there's a good chance you'll see a family of deaf people having a conversation in sign language. Going to the school wasn't just about getting a good education, it was about connecting with a whole new community.

At the school, we didn't really study sign language—that was already my language—but my fluency rocketed because I was using it constantly to communicate with my new friends. Learning nouns and object words is easy in sign language, so I was fluent when it came to having simple conversations about tangible things. It was the concept words that were tricky. "Who," "what," "when," "where," and "why"—the "W" words—can be hard to master at first, because you can't associate them with anything visual. But we worked hard until I had mastered them—I remember sitting at home and watching sign language videos with my parents, fairy tales like "Little Red Riding Hood" and "Goldilocks." I especially loved all the videos with Linda Bove, the deaf actress who played Linda the librarian on Sesame Street. It brought us closer together as a family, having to learn sign language as a team.

Most kids at the school were boarders and stayed in dorms, because their families lived outside of St. Augustine. Around two hundred of us, including me, came home at night after school. I loved being able to go home to my family, and was grateful that my parents had uprooted their lives so that they could be close by.

My favorite times at the school were always those spent playing sports—Little League, city basketball league, soccer, volleyball, you name it. Whatever sport I played, I would figure out what my goals were, and I wouldn't stop working until I achieved them. Sometimes, my friends didn't understand my obsession with winning. Once, at an out-of-state track competition, one of my girlfriends kept bugging me as we were running 'round the track. "You won last week, you gotta let me win this time!" she signed. I didn't get it. I sped off ahead of her and won the gold medal. She won silver. Afterward I found her crying in the bathroom. I told her I was sorry and explained I never meant to hurt anyone's feelings. I just always had an instinctive drive to come in first.

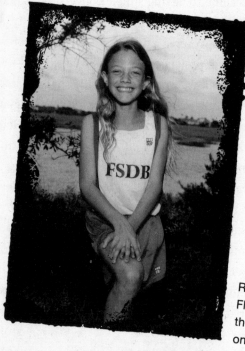

Representing the Florida School for the Deaf and Blind on the track.

Hitting the Amateur Circuit

The second I arrived in St. Augustine, I was racing and training with my dad, even as I was settling into school. A lot of the kids at school had trouble relating to my love for motocross, and there was a fair amount of eye-rolling whenever I would win a trophy or talk about traveling to different states, and later, countries, to race. But that didn't bother me—motocross was in my blood, and I didn't care what anyone else thought.

In Florida the motocross scene is huge, so we were spoiled for choice with races and tracks. Each weekend I would race (this would taper off the older and more experienced I became— I would save my energy for the biggest and most prestigious amateur nationals and qualifier events). At first, the motocross kids were fascinated by me, wondering how I could ride without being able to hear anything. Oh, and then there were their parents: "Isn't it dangerous allowing a deaf kid on the track?" they asked my dad. "Should she even be allowed to ride with the other kids?" They assumed that because I couldn't hear what was going on I'd be a danger to myself and the kids around me. Thankfully at the time I had no idea that anyone wanted me off the track—my parents told me only later. One of the best things about being deaf is that you can't hear anyone talking smack about you.

My parents decided to fight fire with fire—by making me the safest and best girl on the track. Each weekend we would jump in our Coachmen motor home and drive to different tracks. Like Echeconnee Off-Road Park, a rough, loamy dirt track in Georgia. And Hillbilly Hills, also in Georgia. My dad and I spent time working on fundamentals—how to pick my line and keep my line, how to approach turns, how to look for shadows on the ground that indicated a racer was coming up behind me. My senses became heightened, and the bike started feeling more and more like an extension of my body. Every hour I wasn't at school was spent getting me more confident on the bike. Soon enough, the motocross parents back in St. Augustine realized that I was the last thing they needed to worry about. In fact, I was probably one of the safest kids on the track.

Our Motocross Clan

Motocross may not be as huge as basketball or baseball, but once you're involved in the sport, you feel like you're part of a giant extended family, with hundreds of thousands of members. As many as fifty thousand people will attend a pro supercross stadium event, and a crowd of twenty-five to fifty thousand is common at an outdoor motocross national. Even amateur races have a healthy fan base—two hundred or so riders and their families each weekend. It's at the big national amateur events, like the Mini Olympics, which draws six thousand riders from eleven different countries, or Loretta Lynn's, for which twenty-three thousand kids try to qualify, that you get a sense of how big the motocross family really is.

And it's a tightly knit scene. Families will take in other families' kids. Kids will become best friends on the track, and their parents will become best friends off it. Motocross is an expensive sport, so older riders might donate their bikes to younger amateurs. And if a rider is injured, the whole community will try to raise the money to cover medical costs. You'd be surprised how many riders don't have health insurance, so the community sets up foundations—like the RiderDown Foundation—to help friends and family of injured riders deal with medical costs. When sixteen-year-old rider Ricky James was paralyzed from the chest down in 2005, for example, the community held a giant auction, raising $35,000 for him in just one day.

The community exists because we really need each other,

perhaps more so than in other sports. In motocross, kids get paralyzed and kids die—it's a reality. It's a dangerous, expensive, and dirty sport, populated by natural-born rule breakers and risk takers. But the passion that exists among motocross families is second to none. And that's what binds us together.

The Fans

Motocross is particularly known for its loyal and hardy fan base. Oftentimes, they will trek around the country and venture into the near-wilderness just to see a race. Without them, the sport couldn't survive.

The Whoop Monster, for example, is a motocross mega fan. He dresses up in shredded fatigues and carries around a chain saw that he's customized with a horn, attached to the saw's exhaust. You can usually see him at men's motocross races at Spring Creek Motocross Park in Millville, Minnesota. The Whoop Monster says he's the mascot for privateer riders—"privateer" meaning riders with no corporate backing. He even has a customized cart called the Rockin' Whoopmobile that cruises around the track grounds, and he sometimes builds a "Privateer Zone" in the privateer pits, where he hands out drinks, energy bars, and snacks. I only saw him once, at Millville in 2007, and I found him to be hilarious looking. I didn't get the chance to talk to him, though.

Some fans struggle with the notion of women racing dirt bikes—they believe that motocross is a man's sport, all about the hard grind. In the motocross DVD *The Great Outdoors,* one of the mechanics says, "It takes a real man to go thirty-five minutes outdoors." And yes—it does take a real man, *or a real woman,* for that matter. In motocross races you're on the dirt for around thirty minutes, plus two laps, on the gnarliest, roughest tracks out there, often in 100 degree weather. Supercross, on the other hand, is indoors, air-conditioned, and after fifteen laps, you're done. Supercross fans have a seat, a view, and a climate-controlled environment; motocross fans spend their weekends trudging up and down hillsides, sweating. As passionate as motocross fans are about the sport, it's definitely not for everyone.

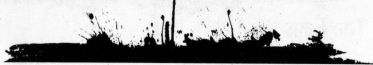

We built a close circle of motocross friends, most of them families with kids that were about the same age as me. There were the Smiths, the Stacys, the Nortons, the Woods, and the Revel brothers, Brian and Brandon. Two years apart in age, Brandon was a year older than me and Brian was a year younger. They were blond-haired, blue-eyed all-American boys and the three of us used to love playing and riding together. Cody Smith and Chad Stacy were my big rivals. I taught the boys some basic signs so we could all communicate with one another, even though there was rarely much need for conversation as we were always either riding or playing some kind of game like football. Yep—I was a classic tomboy.

If there was one thing we would talk about, it would be Loretta Lynn's, the biggest, most prestigious amateur race you can win. The race is held at country singer Loretta Lynn's dude ranch in Hurricane Mills, Tennessee, about an hour away from Nashville. Getting to Loretta's was always the dream, but there were other big national amateur races we wanted to conquer too— like the Spring Nationals at Lake Whitney, Texas; the GNC race in Decatur, Texas; the World Minis in Las Vegas; and the Winter

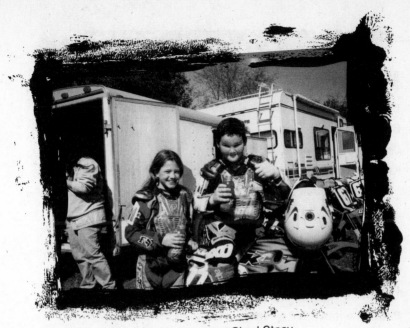

With my friend and competitor Chad Stacy.

Olympics in Gainesville, Florida. And there were the National Motorsport Association nationals—the Branson USA in Galena, Missouri; the Grand National in Ponca City, Oklahoma; and the World Mini Grand Prix in Las Vegas—which aren't quite as prestigious as the others but which I still wanted to win.

As you can gather, nearly all my friends and competitors back then were boys. I was too young to race the women's class, so I ended up racing against boys in the 50 cc, 60 cc, and 80 cc categories, which are for both sexes. ("Cc" refers to the engine capacity—the power of the bike.) I didn't care whether I was racing boys or girls; I just wanted to win. Motocross is a pretty even playing field when you're young. Then boys start getting bigger, and the balance changes—they can handle bigger bikes and have greater upper-body strength. But I had plenty of years of racing boys before I noticed the differences between us.

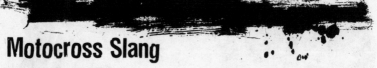

Motocross Slang

Basket case: an old bike that's trashed and doesn't run anymore

Brain bucket: a helmet

Gravity check: a crash

Knobby wheels: the tires on a motocross bike have rubber blocks, or knobs, protruding upward away from the tire to create traction on loose surfaces, so we call them "knobbys"

Pinned: at full throttle, maximum RPMs

Whip: going off a jump, kicking the back end of your bike out to the side, and bringing it back before you land

T-bone: when one rider runs directly into the side of another

Pegs: the footholds where you stand on the bike

Thanksgiving in a Field

There are five big amateur national motocross competitions in America. The first big event is in November—the Mini Olympics (or "Mini O's") in Gainesville, Florida. It is made up of three days of supercross and three days of motocross, and each year the best amateur racers in the world (of all ages) gather at the site, Gatorback Cycle Park, in hopes of becoming the Olympiad Champion. Children as young as four can compete for national attention at this race.

The Mini O's take place over Thanksgiving week, so the first time my family went, in 1999, my mom cooked Thanksgiving dinner in our motor home oven. We cheated a little—she had made pumpkin pies at home ahead of time and packed them for the road, and we grilled a breast of turkey instead of trying to roast a whole Butterball—but still, it was one of those family dinners I'll never forget. As we made more and more friends in the motocross community, our Thanksgivings came to include many hungry mouths, and before long, a whole group of us motocross families would meet annually to eat turkey in a field. It doesn't get much better than that, as far as I'm concerned.

After the Mini O's, there's a long break and then in early March comes the Lake Whitney Spring National, followed by the GNC—the Grand National Championship. For the last few years the GNC has been held at a track called Oak Hill, in Decatur, Texas. The World Mini Grand Prix takes place the following month in Las Vegas—another weeklong affair. Then in July there's Ponca City in Oklahoma, a big warm-up race for the closing race of the amateur season: the Amateur National Championships at Loretta Lynn's ranch. Ponca City and Loretta's are pretty much back-to-back—riders finish up in Ponca City on Saturday and then drive fifteen hundred miles to Tennessee to start practice for Loretta's on Monday morning. Which means living in a field for two weeks or so. In motocross, you literally have to feel at home in the mud. I went to Loretta's for the first time when I was about ten as a spectator—my parents wanted me to see the races there first so that when it was my turn to compete I wouldn't feel intimidated. Even though my folks told me we were there just to have fun, I knew I wanted to return, not as a spectator but as a racer.

Loretta's is the magical bridge between the realms of amateur and professional motocross. Traditionally, boys who are deemed good enough to go pro (normally around the age of sixteen) race Loretta's as their final amateur race. The next race they compete in will be a pro race, an outdoor national. Once they go pro, they do not dip back into the amateur ranks again. Keeping pros and amateurs separate allows amateur boys the breathing room to grow alongside riders of similar ability and experience, rather than having to face off against bigger, more seasoned pro boys. And it makes the transition between amateur and pro much more meaningful. For women, things have always been far less defined. Oftentimes women would go pro

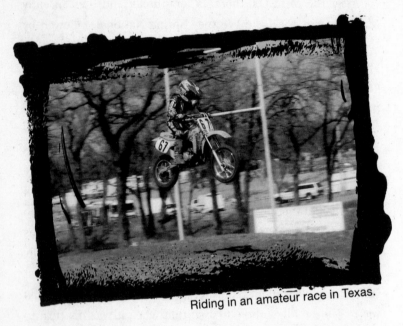

Riding in an amateur race in Texas.

and then continue to race amateur too. Part of the reason was that until 2004, the sanctioning body of motocross (the AMA—American Motocross Association) didn't even recognize women professional racers. That's the reason they could go back and forth—*there were no rules.*

Often the reason pro women stepped back into amateur races was because they weren't being offered the sponsorships, backing, or prize money they deserved in professional races.

So they used amateur races as a source of income. For a long time, that's been the reality in women's motocross. From day one, I felt this wasn't right. First of all, racing against amateurs prevented pro women from being taken seriously. Second, it wasn't fair to the younger amateur girls, having to compete against pro girls. What chance did they stand of winning? More worryingly, this practice fueled the vicious circle of underachievement for women in motocross. To me, it felt like we women were selling ourselves up the river. We should have been pushing for equal prize purses and sponsorship opportunities *as professional racers,* rather than fighting for scraps at the amateur table. This was an issue of self-respect. Early on, my mom, my dad, and I decided that if I was ever to conquer Loretta's, if I was ever going to make a real career out of this, I would go about it in the same way that the boys did—race Loretta's for the last time and then go pro, never returning to amateur racing again. It was time for a new path.

Loretta's—
The Super Bowl of Amateur Motocross

Loretta Lynn's has been held at country singer Loretta Lynn's dude ranch in Hurricane Mills, Tennessee, since 1982, when Davey Coombs Sr. decided to create the ultimate championship for American amateurs (his son Davey Coombs is now one of the biggest promoters in motocross). Loretta herself didn't have any ties to motocross before then—now her name will be forever associated with the sport. The track is rebuilt every year and no one is allowed to ride it before the big event, which attracts more than a thousand top amateur contenders from across the country. Hundreds of motocross families plan their entire summer vacation around it.

Loretta's features thirty-three riding classes based on age, sex, and bike size, with forty-two riders in each class. Almost fourteen hundred amateur riders will compete each year, so it takes a whole week to run the races at Loretta's. When you're not racing, there's plenty to do—dozens of barbecues, games, auctions, and dances, infusing a carnival atmosphere into the whole affair. And if you need to unwind, you can go horseback riding or swim in the creek that runs through the property.

Getting to compete at Loretta's is far from easy. First of all, you have to finish in the top seven or eight at a local qualifier. Then you can move on to the next stage—the regionals. I would usually compete in the southeast regionals, for example, alongside kids from Florida, Alabama, Georgia, and Tennessee. The top riders from each regional get to go to Loretta's—only forty-two per class. So when you line up at the gate, you're lining up alongside the best forty-one riders in the nation for your age group or bike size. That's why Loretta's is such a big deal—you've already gone through a long, arduous filtering process to get to that lineup. After the gate drops, it only takes two and a half minutes to lap the track, but each second is crucial—you'll be racing in front of sponsors, manufacturers, and cameras from cable channels like the Speed Channel and Fuel TV. Loretta's is America's ultimate amateur motocross showcase, just as Davey Coombs Sr. intended, and its winners are expected to become the champions of tomorrow.

Training Day

After my first visit to Loretta's, visions of me winning it immediately began forming in my mind. So my dad started working with me to make my dreams a reality. We started training harder than ever—three days a week at our local track, Pax Trax, and on the weekends we'd head out to Georgia, to our favorite tracks, so I could experience as many different types of dirt as possible. We tried to avoid going to the same place two days in a row.

By this point, my dad and I were already starting to view motocross as something more serious than a hobby. Of course, that affected our relationship. We were no longer just father and daughter hanging out together—we were athlete and coach, with our eyes on a prize. Almost immediately, we started butting heads. To ever have a chance of winning Loretta's requires massive discipline on the part of a racer. You've got to practice fundamentals until you can't even feel your legs anymore. In a typical practice session you're working on left turns and right turns, over and over, figure eights and ovals for hours and hours. Doing that all day long grows unbelievably boring.

One time we were working on technique up in Georgia, while I was still riding a small 65 cc. My dad could tell I was bored.

"Can't we stop?" I signed.

I was tired, hungry, and getting madder every minute. And he knew it. But he said no—we weren't leaving until I'd shown some improvement. I grimaced and revved my engine in frustration. Out of the blue, my clutch popped out, sending me and my bike lunging toward my dad. I mowed him down, and although it doesn't sound very funny, I couldn't stop laughing at the sight of him, wild-eyed, muddy, and furious in the dirt. Even after that, there was no getting out of practicing: my dad refused to let us leave the track until we were done. He was about as grumpy as I had ever seen him and to this day, he jokes that I rammed him on purpose. Of course that's not true, but the point is, there's a lot of blood, sweat, and tears that goes into getting good at motocross.

My dad's an intense trainer and father, and I'm an intense rider and daughter. And my mom, she's all heart too. Life with the Fioleks can be pretty interesting sometimes, and there have definitely been days when everybody has been crying because it's all too much. As things heated up in my career, emotions would really start boiling over. When I was young I deferred to my father on every decision—how to ride, where to ride—but with time I started to have ideas and opinions of my own. I got fed up with having to listen to everything my dad had to say. I was starting to grow up. And very slowly, much in the same way as I had with my deaf friends in Florida, I started to pull away, although it would be years before I would be able to truly detach, and stand alone as a motocross racer.

The Big Crash—and the Great Depression

My first big crash happened during this early period of intense training and racing. I was around ten years old, and we had gone to an amateur race at Daniel Boone raceway in Kentucky, an advanced track for a kid, with jumps that'll make your heart skip a beat. Today, I get a kick out of flying through the air on two wheels, but back then I thought jumps, especially doubles (let alone triples), were plain scary. My dad was trying to help me get over my fear. We both knew that if I was going to get anywhere in motocross, I'd have to get the hang of jumping, and soon.

The day began much like all race days—I signed up in the registration trailer and completed the usual paperwork with my dad. In motocross, race classifications range from A to D, where

D equals "beginner," C equals "novice," B equals "intermediate," and A equals "pro." I signed up for C, novice, and dreamed of the day I could mark the letter A on my sign-up sheet. Before practice started, the riders and their parents were allowed to walk the track and get a feel for it.

"I think you're good enough to try that jump," my dad said, pointing at a giant double in the distance. "Don't be afraid, Ashley."

I looked at the jump and felt flattered that my dad had so much faith in my skills. Because from where I was standing, it looked *gnarly*. I knew that only two or three of the top boys were planning on trying it. Here's the thing with jumps: you don't gain extra points for attempting one, but they will almost always help you gain an advantage. Rolling through a jump is generally going to cost you more time than just flying over it. And there comes a point in motocross where it's dangerous *not* to take jumps. If kids are jumping over your head, there's always a danger that they might land on you. So it's far safer to be flying in the air alongside them. (Interestingly enough, a lot of the pro girls I race with today don't do the jumps. That's primarily because the tracks we ride on and their jumps are designed for pro men. There's one track in Pennsylvania called High Point with really huge jumps—most of the women just rolled over them this year.)

I gazed at the double. If my dad thought I was ready, then I figured, well, I must be ready. I wheeled my new 65 cc bike up to the start gate for the first moto; packed the dirt behind the gate, just like dad had taught me ("You don't want your tires spinning in a trench at the gate," he always told me); and squinted at the double jump one last time. Yep—still gigantic. *Piece of cake!* I thought, trying to convince myself.

Face Plant

The gate dropped and the race began. I rode a steady line, like I always did. Because I can't hear anyone coming up behind me, I'm more restricted in my movements than other riders. The big jump was coming up after the next turn. I hit the gas hard, and soared into the air, jaws clenched. I was flying high—but not high enough, and my bike slammed against the back end of the jump's second mound. POW! My helmet wasn't on my head anymore and I was facedown in the dirt, coughing and spluttering, eating mud and blood all at the same time. I'd just experienced my very first "face plant"—motocross speak for when you crash headfirst. And it wasn't pretty.

I rolled around in the dirt for a couple of minutes, wondering where in the heck my front teeth were. The impact of crashing had knocked me out and my nose was broken. I was having trouble keeping my eyes open and was throwing up all over the place. My body was aching in ways I never knew possible, and I could barely remember my own name.

"Where am I? What's happening?"

The yellow flag went up and I saw my dad come rushing over onto the track. Parents aren't usually supposed to do that—he must have been really freaked out.

"What were you thinking, Ashley! Why did you take that crazy jump?" he signed.

I didn't know what he was talking about. Turns out, earlier on he'd been pointing at a much smaller double jump—not the behemoth that I'd just majorly wiped out on.

My dad kneeled over me, and all color drained from his face. He can't stand the sight of blood—and for a second it looked like *he* might need the paramedics more than I did. "You better take care of your husband," said the doctor to my poor mom, who was trying to look after me *and* stop my dad from being sick on his shoes.

After the paramedics bandaged me up, I made my parents take me back over to the bleachers. Even though I was hurting, I still wanted to watch the other races. But when I went to sit down, everything started spinning. I asked to go back to the motor home. I was in so much pain I couldn't even focus anymore. My mouth was full of gauze and I was still bleeding from cuts and grazes all over my body. Then everything turned black.

I woke up in the backseat of Grandpa Motorcycle's truck, my head on my mom's lap. I was covered in blankets and Mom had this strange look on her face. I guess she was pretty shaken up. We were on the road, headed for the emergency room. When we got there, the doctors kept asking me all these questions, which my dad translated for me, but I couldn't concentrate. I kept falling asleep, sometimes in the middle of a sentence. My mom took a picture of me that day—my nose was broken and puffy, and my lips were bleeding. I still have a scar on my bottom lip where my teeth went through my lip. Not my best look.

The doctors took some X-rays, and I had to have a root canal because my front teeth had been smashed. I was only ten years old and it was all so bewildering, mainly because I didn't understand what was happening. My parents were struggling to find the language to explain what was going on—they didn't know how to sign "root canal," and even if they had, I wouldn't have understood. That was the first time I had to have oral surgery—and believe me, I'll take a broken bone *any day* over oral surgery. When you break a bone the doctors put you in a sling or a cast and then you're done. With this, the dental drama seemed never-ending.

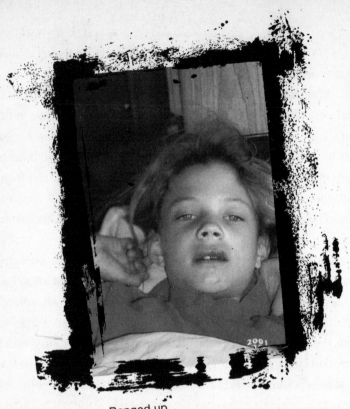

Banged up.

At home my mom had to squirt food in my mouth through a tube. Food is one of my favorite things in the world, so you can imagine what a downer that was having shakes for breakfast, lunch, and dinner. Over a monthlong period we kept having to go back to the hospital so the doctors could decide what steps to take next. That was one of the hardest things for me—I couldn't just move on from the accident. I knew I never wanted to feel this way ever again. For the first time in my life, I was done with motocross.

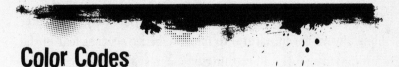

Color Codes

Green: indicates the start of the race

White: one lap to go until the finish

Yellow: caution—when a yellow flag is displayed, competitors must ride cautiously until they have passed the accident or danger that caused the flag

Black with a one-inch white border: disqualification of a rider; that rider must report to the referee at once

Black and white checkered: the end of the race

Red: the race has been stopped due to an emergency situation

Red cross flag: Medical assistance is needed on the track— riders should slow down, and should not try to pass or jump.

Time Out

When I started talking about quitting motocross, my friends and family didn't know what to think. For the first time, I was starting to think about what it must feel like for my parents, having a nutty daughter like me who wanted to jump twenty feet in the air every weekend on a bike that weighed twice as much as she did. I wasn't about to start playing with Barbie dolls or wearing dresses (I think I've worn a dress maybe twice in my life), but I did start looking at other hobbies. My dad bought me a skateboard. I already had a surfboard, and I started using it, even though I'm not crazy about the ocean. I don't really like to swim or go to a lake, or even a swimming pool. A hot tub is about as wet as I usually like to get. Being submerged in water has always felt unnatural to me. Maybe it was that fear of the unknown again . . . I like things you can see and touch, and you never really know what's lurking underwater.

For nearly four months, I couldn't even look at my bike without feeling sick. Then, one day, I realized something. I was *bored*. I started searching deep inside myself and my faith. I have always believed that God has a plan for all of us. Maybe all of this was part of it. Maybe God *wanted* me to experience injury, just like everyone else does in this sport. Maybe God wanted me to know what it felt like to be hurt, so that I could be physically and emotionally prepared for the future.

Faith is a big part of motocross. If you didn't have faith, you probably wouldn't be out there on a bike. It's no coincidence that there are church services at all the big amateur nationals and pro nationals. Every day when I leave my home and go to practice, I ask God to keep me safe, to help me to learn, and to guide and protect me. And whenever I'm on the podium, the first person I thank is God.

Looking back, the period of time following my accident was among the most pivotal in my career—just in terms of figuring things out in my head and getting some perspective on what lay ahead of me. I feel so grateful to my friends and family for their patience and love, for letting me work things out on my own terms. Never did I feel pressure to do anything other than what felt right to me.

One morning, four months after my accident, I tugged on my dad's shirtsleeve. "I want you to teach me how to jump," I signed. We went to Pax Trax and riding my bike again, after such a long break, I realized there was no place for fear in my world. And today, I love the thrill of doubles. Triples—well, I'm not a huge fan; I'll normally take 'em as a double plus a single, thank you very much.

I still have a gray tooth because of that day at Daniel Boone. And it doesn't bother me at all. Every time I look in the mirror it just reminds me not to let fear get in the way of my dreams.

Faith in Moto X

There are always church services before pro races, usually run by Pastor Steve Hudson, who visits the tracks to preach to riders and industry folk. Chappy (as he's known) holds a chapel service at every race after the riders' meeting. He'll go to the hospital when riders are hurt, he'll officiate their weddings, and sometimes he'll even conduct riders' funerals.

It goes back to motocross being a dangerous sport. You hope that someone up there is keeping an eye on you, and lots of people—me included—count on God to keep them safe out there on the track.

My friend and former mechanic Rick Wernli gave me a Bible promise book when he was wrenching for me for a little while. I picked out some things that I read before every race, just seconds before I head to the starting line. Reading the verses makes me feel calm.

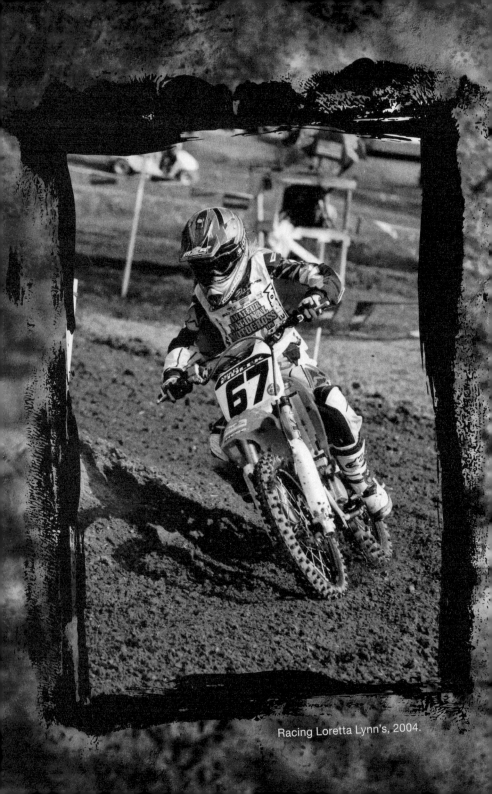

Racing Loretta Lynn's, 2004.

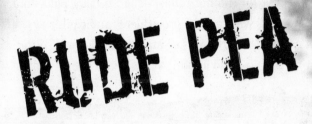

chapter 4

Cheerleaders and Catering?

When I was just a few months old, my mom and dad started calling me Rude Pea—like "Sweet Pea," but with major attitude. The nickname stuck. It was fitting, especially once I started getting into motocross. Off the track, I'm not a fighter—I'm a happy-go-lucky girl who likes shooting goofy YouTube videos with her friends, eating sushi (Philadelphia rolls are my kryptonite), and making banana cream pie. But on the track, it's a different story. If I'm in a race and somebody is messing with me, don't expect me to sit back and take it.

This attitude has served me well in motocross, one of the most macho sports in the world. It's all gasoline, high speeds, and dirt—not what you'd call girly. That's never bothered me, because I've never been very girly myself. But still, there are some people who believe if a girl's on a motocross track, she should be wearing hot pants, posing next to a bike, or handing out energy drinks to the fans. *Cheerleaders and catering*, basically.

And then there are the ads in motocross magazines—sometimes they make my eyes roll right into the back of my head. Companies don't mind using an image of a professional male motocrosser to sell their product, but when it comes to selling women's gear, they prefer to use some hot model in a string bikini. That's great for the hot model—she's getting paid—but what about the girls who are real pro athletes and could use the money? Even as a little girl, I was aware that things were different if you were female—and it didn't sit well with me.

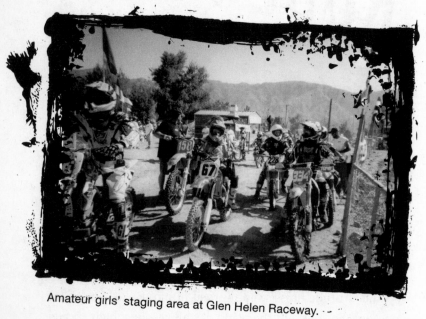

Amateur girls' staging area at Glen Helen Raceway.

There are some people who don't think women's pro racing should exist *at all*. They don't see the point in spending money on seeing girls race because "girls just aren't as fast." Well, they're living in the Dark Ages. Bottom line—girls attract people to motocross who wouldn't otherwise have been interested. The combination of feminine and masculine fascinates the outside observer—"Look at those young girls getting all muddy on these powerful bikes . . . how do they do it?" When a girl is shredding on a dirt bike, it's a sight to behold and always the result of incredible hard work and determination. As has been the case in nearly every sport, women in motocross have had to fight extra hard to be taken seriously, so our stories interest the public at large, a public that might otherwise have ignored motocross.

Fast Friends

In the early days, most of my friends were boys. But in the summer of 2002, when I was around twelve years old, I met two women who would become among my closest friends and allies. Elizabeth Bash—we like to call her E-Bash—started racing when she was twelve years old, and she's just as crazy about motocross as I am. She's four years older than I am, tall (around five foot eight), and a tomboy, a stooge and funnyman all rolled into one, a stoic racer with a taste for pranks. Her relaxed SoCal energy perfectly complemented my hyperactive little self.

I remember when we met, up at the Lake Whitney track in Texas. "How's the track?" she said, looking at her shoes. Actually, like most people, she didn't really talk to *me*. She talked to my parents and had them explain what she was saying to me. I still wasn't that great at lip-reading, and she had no idea how to sign, but I felt a good vibe from her. I'd never had a female friend before who could really relate to my life in motocross and my big dreams. E-Bash was the first member of my motocross sisterhood.

Around the same time, I met Miki Keller—the big mama of women's motocross. She's not actually big in *size*, but she's real big in personality. I had always seen her around at the amateur races and wondered who she was, the lady wearing sneakers

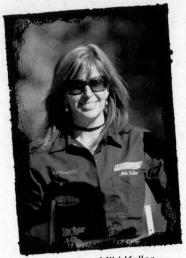

Miki Keller.

with a smudge of mud on her nose. Miki's always running around with her hair up, getting sweaty and dirty, joking around and keeping a sharp eye on things. Miki used to race, so she knows and understands the thrill of riding.

Girl Racers

Women blazed a trail into motocross in the 1960s, competing in long-distance desert races on dirt bikes called Velocettes, B.S.A.'s and Matchless 500s. Until 1975, the women's motocross national championship was known as the "Powder Puff" championship, which didn't sit well with some of the racers, who had to fight long and hard to be recognized as true talents in their sport.

Some of the most memorable characters and pioneers include stuntwoman Tina Clary, who raced against the men in the 1970s and 1980s. Kerry Klied was the first woman to ever hold an AMA Professional Racing License—which was confiscated at a race because the AMA rules did not actually allow for women pro racers. Klied sued, and won, and continued to race professionally against the men. Doreen Payne was the first woman to race against men in a stadium race. She had started out riding BMX bikes and entering competitions as D. Payne so that no one would know she was a girl—she would have been disqualified had they found out her true gender.

In the 1990s, women's professional motocross almost disappeared altogether, with the explosion of ATV racing and the death of a promoter named Mickey Thompson, who had always been an advocate of women's rights in the sport. After he passed away, promoters started refusing to include a women's class in their races, forcing women to compete alongside men or boys in amateur classes. Insulted, many female riders left the sport altogether. Miki Keller founding the WMA, and the recent inclusion of women's motocross in the X Games, brought fresh hope to the survival of women's professional motocross.

And today, if you're a girl who loves motocross, it's up to you to team up with other girls and fight for better rights. Shout loud enough and believe me, the promoters, sponsors, and dealers will listen. Find out how many people it takes to make a rider class, and if you can gather enough girls together, ask your local track promoter to put on a girls-only race. In motocross, if you don't ask, you don't get.

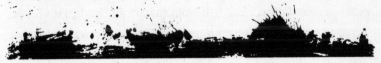

We were finally introduced to Miki at an amateur race at the Cycle Ranch in Texas. At the time, she was heavily involved in the now-defunct Women's Motocross League and was working on starting up a new racing association for women—the WMA, or Women's Motocross Association. Through the WMA, she would fight to keep pro women's racing alive, as there had been talk of removing it from the pro-racing schedule altogether. She looked my dad straight in the eye.

"Ashley's got something special," she said. Then she turned, smiling at me as she held out her hand. "Good to meet you. You're quite a lady." I didn't quite catch what she was saying, because I was too timid to look her in the eye. I was barely twelve years old and still a little shy around people I didn't know, particularly those who couldn't sign. My dad interpreted for me, and I couldn't help but blush at what she had said. I felt something powerful and warm radiating from this lady and had a feeling we would know her for a long time.

Always a go-getter, Miki doesn't have any kids of her own. She says she thinks of the girl riders as her kids. "No one's going to make changes for us," she said at that first meeting. "We have to make them ourselves." Finally, someone *inside* the industry who felt as strongly as we did that women's motocross had to evolve.

The Road to Loretta's

I had grand dreams, but before I was going to bring about my women's revolution, I had to become a better rider. What's more, I had to win Loretta's, or no one would take me seriously. And that meant practice—lots of practice, all over the country.

When I was thirteen, my dad, my mom, and I were out at a track in Tennessee, practicing on my 85 cc bike, working each of the different sections. The track was punctuated with berms, piles of dirt that build up on the outside of a turn. You'll find them on most motocross tracks, and they develop naturally as riders take the same turn over and over again, pushing and piling dirt up with their back wheels until it grows into a wall. I recall the dirt at that particular track was real loamy—meaning a darker-colored dirt with a sticky, viscous feel. I took a five-minute break, peeled off my gloves, and kneeled down, picking up a handful of dirt. I squeezed it, enjoying the way it stayed together in my hands. It wasn't dry, rocky, or sandy—it felt rich and delicious, like chocolate pudding. "It's like Play-Doh," I signed to my dad, and he smiled.

"Good traction," he signed back, nodding.

Most tracks have something called the whoops section, basically a long series of mini-jumps or moguls that you can't really jump. You have to just kind of blast over the tops of them. (The craziest whoops are at the X Games—it is easy to lose control in them, and if you do, you're toast.) The rhythm section, on the other hand, is a series of double or triple jumps. You have to find a good rhythm to get through them smoothly. (I generally prefer a rhythm section over whoops; whoops are gnarly.) That day, I breezed past the whoops section, because I was trying to focus on turns. Turns are where riders shine or lose time.

I was experimenting with how much gas I needed for different kinds of turns, formulating a plan as I made laps around the track—I would take the next corner using a different technique, one that involved bringing the gas back a little later than usual. I was so preoccupied with strategy, I forgot how fast I was going, and before I realized what was happening, I headed straight into a berm. Rather than swerve along its inner contour I plowed straight up its steep side, over the lip, and took off into the air, hitting my brakes frantically as I traveled through the sky. A large murky pond lay on the other side of the berm.

Splash!

Suddenly my bike and I were fully immersed. Motocross gear is pretty heavy and not designed for pond swimming, and I felt its weight drag me down under the tepid, reddish water. In the corner of my eye I saw my parents running over the lip of the berm, waving their arms at me, followed by some family friends who were also at the track. Using all my energy, I slowly heaved myself over to the water's edge, spluttering as I collapsed face-down in the dirt, soaking wet.

Man . . . I hate water! I thought, panting.

I was relieved to be back on land, and as my breathing slowed I became aware of the Georgia sun pounding my back and legs. It was hot—really hot. Burning up, in fact. Then I realized it wasn't the sun that was burning me—hundreds of fire ants had crawled under my gear and were biting the living daylights out of me. I must have crawled out of the pond and lain down right on top of their nest. And they weren't too happy about it—it felt like an entire army of fire ant drones was having a party on my back. (If you've never met a fire ant before, let's just say they're called fire ants for a reason—they *burn*.)

"*They're eating me!*" I signed. My mom, dad, and our friends had gotten to me by this point. My mom launched a rescue mission, ripping off all my gear and brushing the fire ants off of my poor body. Meanwhile our friends' son, who was about my age, was there, watching me get stripped to my riding shorts and tank top as I hopped around in agony. To this day, I cringe when I think about it.

Meanwhile, my dad and his friends were trying to save my bike. They waded in and managed to drag it out of the water. The poor thing looked even worse than I did, covered in red silt. My dad drove it back to the motor home, where he cleaned it lovingly, piece by piece. He even went over it with a hair dryer. Both the bike and I made a full recovery, I'm pleased to say.

Blountville, Tennessee

Another time I was at a track called Muddy Creek in Blountville, Tennessee, for a Loretta Lynn's regional qualifier. I was competing in the boys' 65 cc class. We headed out to the track to practice before the race, and my dad and I were overwhelmed by what we saw. A sea of helmets, bikes, and boys, so many, in fact, you could barely see the dirt. "I'm not sure about this, Ashley," my dad signed. "There are too many boys out there . . . this is insane." I felt apprehensive but shrugged my shoulders. "I *have* to. It's a qualifier," I signed.

I rolled up to the gate and took off into the fray. Within seconds, the madness engulfed me—I saw a boy go down in front of me, his bike skidding in the dirt. To my left were riders, to my right were riders—there was nowhere for me to go except forward, and into the boy's bike. My front wheel collided with his and the impact propelled my body over the handlebars. I flew into the air, landing square on my elbow. A dull pain overwhelmed my entire arm and I felt too weak to move, despite the rush-hour traffic zooming all about me. I knew I was screaming because my mouth was open and my lungs were working overtime. The blur of colors, the gas fumes, the dirt in my mouth overcame me. It felt like I was drowning.

The yellow flag went up. I couldn't feel my arm until I tried to move it—then shooting pain like shards of glass reminded me that it was still there. X-rays later showed I had broken my humerus. This was my *very first broken bone,* but I didn't cry. I very rarely cry when I break bones.

That said, the ride to the hospital was a nightmare—the road was uneven, and each bump seemed to rebreak the bone, over and over again. When we got to the hospital the doctors gave me something to numb the pain—morphine, I think. There was a documentary on the TV in my room about dinosaurs, and in my haze I remember laughing at the images so hard my chest hurt. This was my first experience of painkillers and their strange side effects. My parents watched me cry with laughter as the doctors put my arm in a sling. They thought I was losing my mind.

"Are you OK, Ashley?" they signed. And that made me laugh even harder.

I knew it was tough on my folks, watching me get bashed up all the time. My mom is always up in the stands watching, and whenever I crash she counts to ten slowly to see if I get up. If I do, and if my dad is with me, she keeps her cool. She knows that running down and acting hysterical won't solve anything. But if I don't get up off the ground, she always runs onto the track to make sure I'm not concussed or anything.

After breaking my humerus in Blountville I was in a sling for a couple months. I couldn't race, of course. I couldn't even ride my 65 cc—it was impossible to hold on. Not being active was torture for me. I passed the dull hours the best I could, making videos and watching television. Sitting still for that long is unnatural for me. But there was no talk of quitting riding this time. I had already been through that before, after my crash at Daniel Boone. By now, I was 100 percent sure my future lay in motocross.

Even when, later on, I broke my left collarbone *and* my right wrist—*at the same time*—I still didn't doubt my chosen path in motocross. That crash took place at the 2003 Loretta Lynn's regional qualifier at Paradise Valley MX in Georgia. The doctors had to put both my arms in a sling, and for six weeks life was really awkward, mainly because I couldn't use my hands to sign. My hands are my voice—so not being able to use them was like someone had put duct tape over my mouth.

Luckily, my mom and dad can understand me the way I talk, although it takes most people a little while to get used to it. My voice sounds different from most people's because I had to learn how to use it without ever actually knowing what speech sounds like. Sometimes people seem embarrassed when I try talking to them, because they can't understand what I'm saying. That's OK, it just takes a little time to get used to it, I tell them. Sometimes I sing real loud, just to annoy my mom. Even though I can't hear myself I'm pretty sure I won't be winning *American Idol* any time soon.

I had already raced a different regional qualifier for Loretta Lynn's two weeks before the accident, so at least I made it through. In 2003, I was finally going to race Loretta Lynn's, alongside the best kids in the country—albeit with my new set of injuries. I knew I wouldn't be breaking any records at Loretta's, not with a broken wrist and collarbone. Nonetheless, I insisted on competing. Loretta's for me was about more than winning, it was about the feeling it gave me, being surrounded by so many motocross kids from all over the country. The feeling of belonging, and the electricity generated by so many hopes and dreams concentrated in one field in rural Tennessee. For that, there's nothing quite like Loretta's. I went ahead and raced with my barely healed broken collarbone and wrist, finishing in an abysmal twenty-second place, in a bunch of pain, with a smile on my face. There was always next year to prove myself.

Born into Motocross

Just as 2003 was drawing to a close, God sent us a very special gift—Kicker, my baby brother. People ask if that's his real name—it is. A kicker is an unexpected bump in the track that can send you and your bike flying. And he kicked up a storm in my mom's belly for nine months before he came out, blond, blue eyed, and vocal. Unlike me, he could hear just fine. The day before he was born, we were at a track, practicing, and within five days, my mom and my new baby brother were back in the motor home and on the road, headed for a race. As a family, we were on a mission—a motocross mission—and now Kicker was part of it too.

After my brother arrived, my dad decided it was time to retire the old Catalina and invest in a new motor home—a Four Winds Chateau. It felt giant compared to the old RV, and deluxe. It had a generator, so it always had power. I'd get up in the morning when we were on the road and take a hot shower and my mom would cook breakfast—it was just like being at our real home. There was a refrigerator and a couch and a TV—even a separate bedroom at the back. For once, we wouldn't all have to sleep in the same room. We'd long ago forgotten the meaning of the word "privacy," but I felt like it might do my parents some good to get some alone time, even with little tiny Kicker crying up a storm in the bedroom at night.

My mom, Roni—what a trouper. Out of all of us, she's prob-ably sacrificed the most. My dad and I would be out in the field having fun, and she'd be taking care of Kicker and hanging out in the motor home. Motocross races tend to involve lots of walk-ing and climbing—it's a real rugged sport, whether you're a racer or a spectator; now imagine doing that with a newborn baby. There's no glory being a mom at a motocross national, and the spotlight was always on me—but my mom just took it all on. She was so unselfish about everything, looking after us all while we chased my motocross dream.

One day she handed me a spoon and told me to talk into it. "It's your microphone and I'm going to interview you," she signed. I looked at her like she was crazy. "So, Ashley Fiolek, how does it feel to be the Loretta Lynn's champion this year?" she continued, looking at me intently. I couldn't stop laughing, but my mom was dead serious. "Sweetie, you better be prepared, because one day that spoon is going to be a real microphone, and you better know what you're going to say!"

Sarah Whitmore—My Partner in Grime

Pro racer Sarah Whitmore had always been a hero of mine, from the time I was really little. Today, I'm lucky enough to call her my best friend and confidante. Around five foot eight and seven years my senior, Sarah is the older sister I never had. She has long golden hair and warm brown eyes and is real pretty, like a fairy godmother almost—she's one of those beautiful-inside-and-out kind of girls.

We didn't get to meet until 2004 at Glen Helen, a famous track in California. I was there for amateur day and I guess she had seen me race a couple of times. She approached my dad in her easy, friendly way, and I couldn't believe it—was Sarah Whitmore talking to *my* father? She was one of the best girl pros around, a top girl in the WMA, and a seasoned Loretta Lynn's champion. Sarah was in the holy trinity of female riders, the ones who always seemed to be talked about in the press—Sarah Whitmore, Tarah Gieger, and a girl called Jessica Patterson. All three would come to play an important role in my motocross life, in very different ways.

Sarah asked my dad all the usual questions that everybody asks about me—like, how do I know when to shift, how do I stay aware of what's happening around me on the track? I was so shy and starstruck, I just shuffled my feet in the earth and could barely say a word. My dad and I exchanged e-mail addresses with her and promised to stay in touch.

Later that year, Sarah and I ended up at the same Loretta Lynn's qualifier in Ohio. She was racing the women's class, and I was racing the nine-through-thirteen girls' class. The night before the qualifier, we hung out for the first time without my parents and got to know each other a little better. We talked in my parents' trailer—or communicated the best we could, bearing in mind she had no prior experience of conversing with deaf people. She seemed to take a genuine interest in my opinions and what I had to say, so I tried teaching her some sign language. We had a pen and paper, and I showed her the whole alphabet and explained how to construct simple phrases.

"What do you wanna learn to say?" I asked her, watching her lips so I could understand her answer.

"Hmm . . . I think you should teach me how to say 'cute boy' in sign language," she giggled. "I think that's very important." We both collapsed with laughter. My shyness had disappeared.

Knowing that someone like her was paying attention to me—even though I was deaf—made me walk a little taller from that moment on.

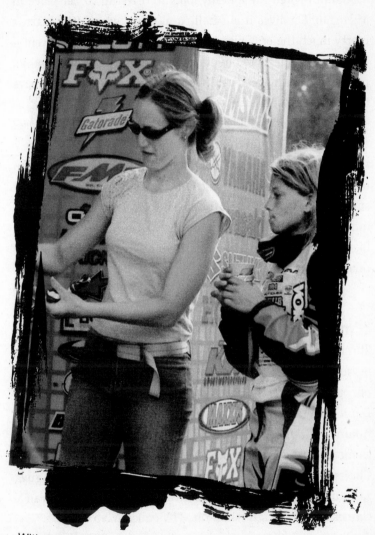

With Sarah Whitmore at Loretta Lynn's in 2004.

She introduced me to a bevy of sponsors and went around singing my praises to whoever would listen. "Watch out for Ashley, she's going to win! Just you wait and see!"

Sarah invited me and my folks to drive up to her place in Michigan. She lives in a small rural town, where Wal-Mart is pretty much the only place to hang out if you're under twenty-one. We went in there one time and I started messing around, pointing at the biggest stereo in the electronics section. "I have that," I signed to Sarah.

"Really? That's cool," she responded, doing her best to form the words with her fingers.

I started cracking up. "Not really . . . I'm deaf—duh!" I love to make fun of my deafness, and sometimes that takes people by surprise. One of my favorite pranks is to grab a friend's iPod, put in the earphones, and dance around like a maniac, pretending like I can hear the music. Sometimes a sense of humor is all it takes to forget life's problems.

"I'm Gonna Kick Your Butt, Travis Pastrana!"

Through motocross I have met a lot of interesting and unique personalities, and made a lot of good friends: Sarah and E-Bash of course, but also Ronnie Renner, a freestyle motocross rider; Daniel Dhers, a BMX rider (whom I dated very briefly); Lyn-Z Adams Hawkins, a skateboarder; and Travis Pastrana, an extreme sports hero who won the World Freestyle Motocross Championship when he was fourteen, was one of the first guys to figure out how to do backflips on a motorcycle, and hosts an X Games–meets–*Jackass* show on MTV called *Nitro Circus*.

Travis and I became friends in the spring of 2004 at a track called Hangtown near Sacramento. I was with Sarah and we were all playing around on the go-karts. Sarah was dating Travis at the time. I guess I was in a feisty mood because the first thing that came out of my mouth when I met him was:

"I'm gonna kick your butt, Travis Pastrana!"

Not everyone understands me when I speak, but he did. I think he thought it was the funniest thing he'd ever heard, this little deaf girl giving him beef on the go-karts. Of course, I said it with a smile on my face. It's funny how much attitude I had, especially compared with how shy I used to be. Motocross had transformed my entire personality. The more I pushed myself on the bike, the less fearful I became of the world in general. Where I used to be quiet around people I didn't know, now I love nothing more than goofing around in front of hearing kids, giving autographs, and pulling pranks.

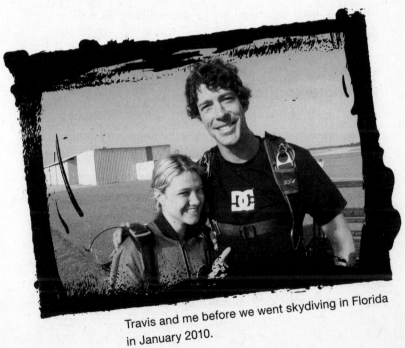

Travis and me before we went skydiving in Florida in January 2010.

Travis comes down to Florida every winter to ride, so after we met, we started hanging out for a couple of days each time he was around. One time we went to Pax Trax, and it was the first time he and I had ridden together on a regular track. He was riding an older trail bike and he was having trouble keeping up with me—I had just graduated to a 125 cc. He told me later he was really embarrassed that I had outpaced him. Which I loved, of course.

Travis and I are natural pranksters—and sometimes it gets extreme. One time he came at me with his clutch and throttle wide open. He'd forgotten that I'm deaf and figured I'd hear him coming and get out of his way. By the time I saw him hurtling toward me, it was too late—we crashed and both went flying over a berm. Afterward everyone was looking at him like he was crazy for taking out a fourteen-year-old girl. I shrugged and gave him a big high five. "It's OK," I signed, laughing. "I would have done the same."

Rolling with the Regals

Before Loretta Lynn's in 2004, my family took me on the road for five weeks to train with our friends the Regals in Michigan. Like us, the Regals are 100 percent committed to the sport. Two of their kids, Kyle and Casaundra, wanted to be pro racers, so their parents did everything in their power to make that happen. Kyle turned pro in August 2009.

The Regals' track was groomed so that it mimicked Loretta's, right down to the real deep ruts. Mark Pelligrino, Kyle and Casaundra's stepdad, was training us, and he didn't put up with any nonsense from us kids—it was his program, or you were out! The fact that he put so much work into training someone else's kid tells you a little bit about how the motocross community works.

We trained every single day for five weeks, and at the end of it, I was ready.

Honky Tonkin'

Leading up to the 2004 race at Loretta's, I had to work hard to keep myself calm. I had been among the top riders at the Loretta's qualifiers and had put in a consistently strong performance all year. I couldn't *wait* to show everybody what I could do, especially after 2003's nonperformance. I knew there was going to be plenty of competition, but I also had a feeling this could be my year. I felt giddy dreaming so big—I'd never won a title before, but now here I was hoping to take the biggest one of them all. Ricky Carmichael, Jeremy McGrath, Travis Pastrana—all the big guys had won at Loretta Lynn's before hitting the big time. My dad and I had put too much work in, broken too many bones, spent too many hours in the dirt, for things not to go my way. And after five intense weeks of preparation at the Regals', nothing seemed impossible.

We arrived at Loretta Lynn's that Saturday and drove by a sign at the entrance that reads NO TRESPASS'N. It always makes me chuckle. Loretta Lynn's Ranch is much more than a home for a famous honky-tonk singer—it comes complete with an RV park, log cabins that you can rent, a swimming pool, a recording studio, and a concert pavilion. There are no less than three museums on the site—the eighteen-thousand-square-foot Coal Miner's Daughter Museum, the Grist Mill Museum, and Loretta's Doll and Fan Museum, filled with her collection of antebellum dolls.

When we arrived the RV park was already filling up with

fans, racers, and their families. I saw a bunch of my friends hanging out, including Sarah. She was by herself, wrapped in a blanket, and wasn't smiling. I ran up to her to find out what was wrong.

"Don't hug me!" she signed, and held her hands out, blocking my way. I stopped in my tracks, and my heart fell. Had I done something wrong? Sarah smiled weakly. "I'm sick," she signed. "You can't come too close."

She wrote down on a piece of paper "Epstein-Barr virus," and I ran and showed it to my parents. It sounded frightening.

"Epstein-Barr . . . that's like mono, isn't it, Jim?" said my mom. She explained to me as best she could that Sarah was going to be OK but that she had a kind of flu that doesn't really go away for a long time and makes you weak. I felt so bad for her. I spent as much time with Sarah as I could when I wasn't practicing. Sometimes she'd sleep and I'd go take a swim in the creek. It was hot, sticky, and humid, so I jumped off a little cliff into the creek and splashed around.

Before the qualifiers in March, we had received some good news—there would be a change in the way the classes were structured this year. Before, girls aged nine through fifteen were racing one another. Now they had dropped the maximum age to thirteen—my age at the time—which filtered out some of the older, bigger girls from my race.

We had to race three motos on three separate days; each was fifteen minutes long, plus two additional laps. The track was gnarly—a simple layout but mulchy and rutted. The weather was on my side and my body felt energized by the crowds. I saw my mom waving on the sidelines. Sarah was run-down, but well enough to announce the girls' races. I hoped to make her proud.

Around me, forty-one of the best motocross teenagers in

America revved their engines—I couldn't hear it, but I felt the vibrations in the air and inhaled the exhaust fumes. Then the starting gate fell backward and we sped into the dirt. I got the holeshot (motocross speak for being the first rider around the first turn) and pushed ahead. I kept my line and opened up the throttle, remembering what my dad had taught me about leaning into the turns, when to open up the throttle, how to position my body. The silence in my head allowed me to concentrate fully on everything that was going on around me—it was as though I had eyes in the back of my head. No one was getting past me, and I felt completely at ease. It was only as I crossed the finish line in first place that I started feeling nervous. Only one-third of the battle was won.

Who's That Deaf Girl?

Two days later, a small crowd had gathered to watch the second moto. Word had spread about the "deaf girl." I was a little nervous this time around—the sky was an ominous gray and it looked like it might rain any minute. The last thing I needed was a muddy track. Mud racing is like Russian roulette—no matter how skilled you are, no matter how well prepared, the mud will trip you up when you least expect it. It might even creep into your engine and leave your bike a steaming wreck on the sidelines. In motocross they call mud "the great equalizer"—a deceptively deep puddle can topple the greatest rider and allow lesser racers to win. Luckily, the clouds cleared right before we lined up at the gate, and I relaxed a little.

I got a great start and took the holeshot again, but this time my good friend Lindsay Myers was on my back. We were neck and neck around each turn, battling it out for first place. But I had determination on my side, and it pushed me to the finish line a comfortable distance ahead of her.

Afterward my dad and I were in the pit going over the race and Lindsay walked up to me, helmet in hand. "No hard feelings?" I signed, my dad interpreting for me. She shook her head and gave me a huge hug. Life's too short for hard feelings in motocross. We all understand the need to win.

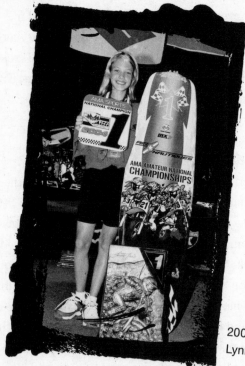

2004 Loretta Lynn's Champion.

Two days later was the third and final moto. This time nearly two thousand people were watching this race, dotting around the fringes of the sprawling track, hanging out on the dirt, waiting to see if the deaf thirteen-year-old girl from Florida would actually make it home with the trophy. I saw families sitting with their coolers and their sun chairs and noticed that a crowd of about a hundred people had already gathered around the podium, waiting to congratulate whoever ended up winning this trophy.

The gate dropped, and I was gone! I got the holeshot again, and this time there was no beating me—I was so confident and so determined to win. As I flew over the finish line in first place I punched the air. I saw Sarah on the sidelines, and knowing she had seen me win Loretta's made me feel doubly proud.

Before I knew it, my mom and my dad were next to me, helping me get my helmet off and hugging me. I saw Sarah run up to the announcer's tower—she wanted to make sure they said my name right. "It's pronounced Fy-lek, not Fee-oh-lek," she told them. The winner's trophy was gigantic, like a big piece of rock with a big "Number 1" carved into it. The grandstand was outside, in the same spot where Loretta Lynn always sings whenever she holds concerts on her property. It's a big stage and all our friends, family, and fans were sitting in rows, watching as we got our awards and were interviewed. My dad jumped up on the stage to interpret for me. The race announcers didn't understand what he was doing at first—they had no idea I was deaf. I had been going to Loretta's for four years, and this was the first time I had won anything there. More than anything, this felt like affirmation that I was on the right path. All our hard work was starting to pay off.

We had to hurry back to Florida afterward—I had school on Monday and had already missed a week of classes. So there was barely any time to celebrate, aside from stopping at a Chinese restaurant for some crab wontons (my favorite). As we rolled back into St. Augustine, me a Loretta's champ, I had a feeling things were going to be different from now on.

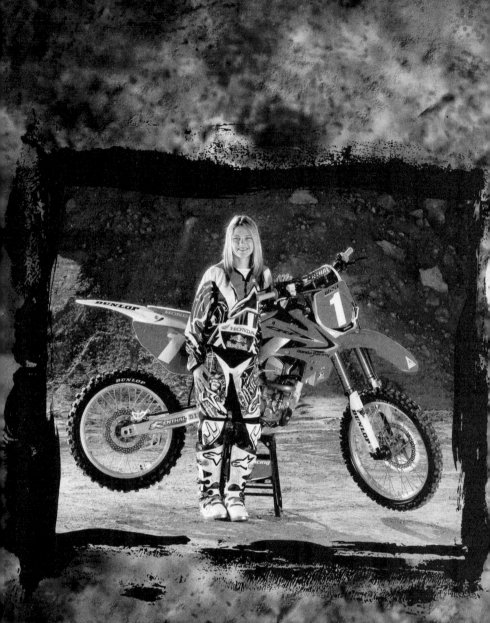

that year, was surprised to learn that I was deaf. Keith called Bill Savino—the man in charge of American Honda's amateur program—and convinced him to come and watch my third moto. Afterward, Keith and Bill both caught up with my father. "We'd *love* to help Ashley out," they said. Neither my dad nor I knew what they meant by that exactly, but we were thrilled by the attention.

A few months later, on a regular weeknight evening, the phone rang at our house in St. Augustine. My dad picked up—it was Bill Savino on the other end. I remember popping my head into the family room. My dad was pacing around, as he always does when he's talking business on the phone. "We'd like Ashley to be part of our amateur program and part of American Honda," Bill told him. They wanted to supply me with bikes and parts (they gave me two Honda CR85s). And most important, manufacturer support was always the first real step toward a professional career.

Immediately after hanging up, my dad grabbed my mom and me, sat us down, and shared the good news.

Excitement welled up in my chest, tempered by a sense of bewilderment. Things were happening so quickly. It felt surreal. Watching my parents' animated faces, their lips and hands moving at hyper speed, I felt oddly distant from it all. *Just keep working, keep racing, keep winning,* I reminded myself. Those were things I could understand perfectly well.

Going to Japan

Each year, the American Motocross Association (AMA) would send the two top girls from Loretta's to the All Japan Motocross Championship. In it, top amateur women from ten different countries were invited to race against the best Japanese riders, on one of the biggest tracks. The competitors had such great

chapter 5

ACCELERATION

Hello, Honda

When I was a little girl I always dreamed of being the number one girl in the world and riding a factory Honda bike—a prototype bike, at the absolute cutting edge of motorcycle technology. Being a factory racer was an honor given to only a handful of the very best riders in the world—*all of them men*. I longed to be the first woman in American history to join the ranks of a factory team, the ultimate motocross fantasy. I wasn't quite there yet, but after my performance at Loretta's, Honda (one of the "Big Four" motorbike manufacturers, alongside Yamaha, Suzuki, and Kawasaki) did cast a glance my way.

Keith Dowdle from American Honda happened to be in the crowd at my first moto at Loretta Lynn's. Impressed, he returned to see how I did in the second. After watching me win again, he sought my father out. "She's very good," he told my dad. "Let's see how she does in the next moto!" He too, like so many at Loretta's names—Larissa Papenmeier, Elien de Winter, Saya Suzuki. I went with my dad, who would become my international chaperone in years to come (my mom would normally stay home and hold down the fort with Kicker). This would be the first overseas trip I had ever made, and likewise for my father. It marked the start of my new life as a frequent flyer.

Our flight to Japan, from Jacksonville via Atlanta, took a good sixteen hours. My dad and I decided we should try to stay awake for the whole flight. That way we'd be on the same clock as the Japanese when we arrived. By the time we touched down in Tokyo I was not only exhausted, but a ball of nerves. I was only thirteen, one of the youngest girls to be invited. Was I out of my depth, agreeing to race against all these riders with exotic names from around the planet?

"They wouldn't have invited you if they didn't think you were good enough!" my dad reminded me, and I knew he was right.

All we wanted to do after landing was get some food and pass out. The hotel had given us coupons for a complimentary dinner in the lobby restaurant, so we decided to take advantage of them and I ordered a steak, a classic Ashley favorite. In my quasi-delirious state, everything seemed funny—especially the steak once it arrived. It was the thinnest little thing I had ever seen in my life, about as wide as a quarter. "I guess they don't have much room for cows around here?" my dad signed, and I could have died laughing.

The next day we took a bus with all the other motocross racers to Sendai, a city in northeastern Japan. The FIM had arranged a luncheon to welcome us and I was giddy with excitement, not only to spend time in the same room as all these incredible riders, but also to try the weird and wonderful foods at the buffet table.

The next day a bus came to the hotel to pick us up and take us to the track. Tons of media and fans greeted us as we arrived, taking photos of us as we got off the bus. I felt like Hannah Montana. I had never had so many people wanting to meet me before—or any other female motocrosser. My dad and I exchanged raised eyebrows—I guess we weren't in Kansas anymore.

Thumbelina

The race was at Sportsland SUGO, one of the biggest motorsports facilities in Japan, with a spectator capacity of fifty thousand. As we wandered around the track I noticed that the media folks were pointing and laughing at me. I asked my dad to find out why. "Apparently it's because you're so small," he told me. "They can't believe you're racing against all these bigger girls." I was probably four feet five inches tall and was riding a little Honda CR85 at that time. The president of the FIM's motorcycle division in Japan told us that for the race, I would be riding a big-wheel bike instead, which lifts you three inches higher off the ground than a regular sixteen-inch wheel. Apparently all the other girls would be racing big wheels.

"But we don't ride a big wheel," my dad said. "We ride the standard wheel."

He laughed. "It's OK, why don't you just try it? It'll be fun."

"We're not here to have fun," said my dad. "*We're here to win.*"

No one really believed we meant business until we lined up for the race qualifier the next day, sixty of us girls, from Japan and around the world. Saya Suzuki, the Japanese champion, was expected to win. As for me, everyone had discounted me because of my size. But as soon as the gate dropped, they reevaluated. I had been nervous, but my dad's faith in me had erased any self-doubt I may have had, and I pushed forward ahead of most of the girls, into fourth place. I passed Elien de Winter, a well-known mini rider, and made what some Japanese commentators later called "an aggressive pass" on one of their champions. I caught up to Saya Suzuki, and by the end of the race I was right on her back wheel. I finished just inches behind her. No one could believe this tiny deaf girl on her 85 cc bike had come so close to beating the mighty Saya Suzuki.

That night, during dinner, it started to rain. And by the time we got back to the track the next day, it was a muddy mess. I didn't fare quite so well in the race this time. Slipping and sliding in the quagmire, I crashed a few times and wound up finishing in eleventh place—still not a bad result, but not as newsworthy as my second place the previous day. "Don't worry, Ashley," my dad said. "Anything can happen in a mud moto. It's not your fault." In the end, Saya Suzuki ended up winning for Japan.

On the plane back to Florida, I was still buzzed from my experience. I didn't fully appreciate that this was going to become a way of life for me—traveling the world and experiencing different cultures. I couldn't wait to tell my friends at school about it all—the skinny steak, how I almost beat Saya Suzuki, and how we were treated like rock stars at the racetrack. But my stories fell on deaf ears (pardon the pun!). "Oh, who cares, Ashley," said one of my friends. Most of them reacted the same way—they didn't want to know.

I did have a couple friends from FSDB who would occasionally watch me race or spend weekends up in Georgia when I trained. But at the end of the day, no one really understood why I thought dirt bikes were so cool. It was a hard lesson for me to learn—the kids I had spent the last eight years with at school, from 1998 until 2006, couldn't relate to the most important thing in my life.

Not long after I returned from Japan, in the middle of ninth grade, I stopped going to FSDB. I had already been missing so many classes because of my schedule—it had gotten to the point of "go to school, or ride." My closest bonds at that time were with hearing people in motocross, not my deaf friends at the school. So it wasn't a difficult choice. My parents started homeschooling me, and it felt like a weight lifted from my shoulders.

In hindsight, I think pulling away from my deaf life at that point was all about my search for identity. Since then, I've come full circle—I am just starting to become involved in the deaf community again, and likewise, the deaf community has just started to take an interest in me. But at that point in my life, leaving school was a statement I had to make—not just to my friends, but to myself. "This is me—motocross is what I am," I told Mandy, one of the few friends at the school who had tried to understand my obsession with motocross. "I am doing this because, one day, I am going to be a professional motocross racer. My mom and dad believe in me, even if no one else does."

For years, my parents had been balancing my school schedule and my race schedule. I hated having to pick which races to do; now I could compete in them all. I committed to a life on the road, a life with no routine or certainty, where pain and injury lurked around every turn—but it was the life that I felt happiest leading. We planned to have me race about fifteen times a year—less than many amateur motocrossers—but eight of those races would be amateur nationals, the most prestigious races in the country.

Now that I didn't have to go to school, I was able to focus totally on my motocross program. I would start my day with an hour of cardio training. Then some schoolwork. Then I'd spend hours doing fundamentals on the track, followed by the gym for strength training and more homework. When I was at FSDB, I was able to stay in shape by joining the cross-country and track teams. Now that I was homeschooled, I had to develop my own fitness regime. We consulted a few different trainers, who came up with tailor-made fitness schedules for me, incorporating daily cardio and strength-training exercises. I became very good friends with my stationary bike at home and our rowing machine. And when we were on the road, my trainer, Robb Beam, would be on the other end of the phone with advice on how and where to exercise. Running up and down any available staircase, for example.

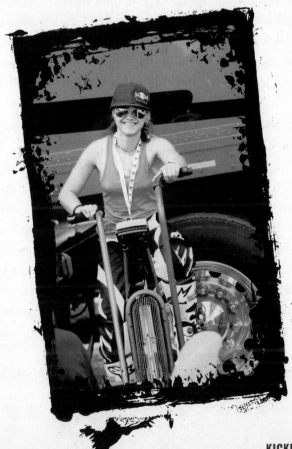

Warming up
for a race.
Carl Stone

The WMA Is Born

Just as my career was starting to take flight, Miki's hard work behind the scenes was beginning to pay off. In 2004, out of the ashes of the Women's Motocross League, she founded the WMA, the Women's Motocross Association, a sister body to the AMA. Technically the AMA was supposed to represent both men and women, but for the longest time the AMA wouldn't recognize women as professionals or offer a women's professional class. Under the WMA, Miki could create a women's pro class and manage all women's pro racing.

With Miki in charge, we knew opportunities for women were going to start opening up. She had a good track record—she had guided the career of Heidi Henry, America's first female freestyle motocrosser, whom she persuaded to freestyle when no other women were. She's helped girl racers get on ESPN and has gotten them featured in women's magazines that wouldn't normally touch motorcycles with a ten-foot pole. Miki rides too, for fun—but working on behalf of young female riders like me is probably a full-time job.

Getting women's pro racing fully recognized has been an uphill battle. And she'll have to start from scratch to get pro women indoors for supercross (the only times girls get to race supercross is at the X Games) since supercross promoters tend to have the same attitudes that many of the outdoor motocross promoters used to have. In case I haven't already mentioned it, this isn't a girls' scene. Not all the other girls are interested in this side of things—the business side, the PR side, getting the exposure necessary to grow our side of the sport. For me, it's crucial. Yes, winning is important—but so is making this sport more balanced.

Stefy Bau, a pro racer from Italy who gave me lots of good

advice between the years of 2003 and 2005, urged my dad and me to stick to our mission. "When you become a pro, make sure you get paid by sponsors," she told him. "Don't just settle for free product. That will help women's motocross grow—if everybody sticks together and demands the same things." Her words have stayed with me and my dad to this day.

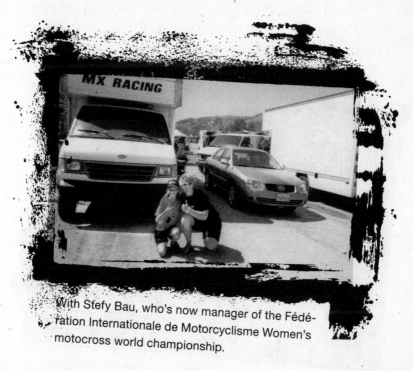

With Stefy Bau, who's now manager of the Fédération Internationale de Motorcyclisme Women's motocross world championship.

Once I went pro, that would be it—*no more amateur racing*, no matter how tempting the cash rewards were. We believed the two should be kept separate, so that amateur kids could get a chance to shine and the sport as a whole could grow for women. That's why we had to think very carefully about when I was going to finally go pro—the timing had to be just right.

"A Lot of Work, a Lot of Money— a Lot of Everything"

Between 2004 and 2007 I raced pretty much all the amateur nationals, trying my best and winning as many as I could. In all I took home twelve more national championships and became one of the top girls in girls' amateur motocross. I won the GNC, the Lake Whitney Spring Classic, the World Mini Grand Prix in Las Vegas, the Mini Olympics, and the Ponca City National Championship. Most of them more than once.

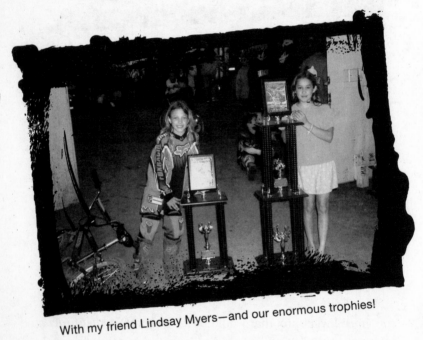

With my friend Lindsay Myers—and our enormous trophies!

In 2005, we went to a track called TMT in Tennessee to train for Loretta's. I had high hopes of another win that year—there was no reason I shouldn't. Then in the first weekend of training I came off my bike hard—so hard I was knocked out. I was carried off the track and taken to the hospital. When I came to, my parents sat me down and tried to explain to me what had happened, but every time they told me anything, I forgot it a second later. The effects of the concussion lasted for a couple hours. In addition, I had separated my AC joint—basically, I separated my shoulder blade from the collarbone. The doctors told me I'd be out of action for "quite some time."

"No way," I said. "*I have to race.*"

I took a week off and got back to training. I didn't care what anyone said. There was no way I was missing out on Loretta's because of an injury.

Because I was fourteen years old at this point, I had graduated into the women's class—which meant I'd be racing against big 125 and 250 motorcycles on my little 85. Most of the other girls were older than me—aged sixteen to twenty-two. I ended up in seventh place overall, and as far as we were concerned, it was actually a great result. The six girls ahead of me all had WMA pro licenses and in spite of my injury, I was the first amateur to cross the finish line. So the way my family saw it, I was the winner.

You'd think that after winning Loretta's, getting support from Honda, and winning all these amateur races, money would have started rolling in. Strangely enough, the more success I enjoyed, the tougher things became—emotionally *and* financially. Yes, we were getting all this free stuff—free motorcycles, free parts, and free gear—but suddenly I was feeling all this pressure to appear at every single amateur race. Before, we were only hitting one or two of them each season, maybe. Now we had to be on the road, away from home, for weeks on end or risk losing support from the industry the following year. So all the money we *thought* we'd be saving by getting free bikes and gear went straight back into my program, paying for gas, and keeping us on the road.

My dad was somehow managing to work his job as a software developer for a health insurance company in Jacksonville on top of being my coach. The house needed work, of course, because we'd been on the road for so long, and both my parents drove beat-up trucks. Yep—we were *broke*, overspending on travel costs and living paycheck to paycheck. Some of my parents' friends were ba⊠ ed—why would we put ourselves through the hardship?

"It's like training an Olympic athlete," my mom would say to anyone who thought we were crazy, living the life we did. "It's a lot of work, a lot of money—a lot of everything. But it's our way of life, and we love it."

Money

Amateurs don't win any prize money, not even if they win Loretta's. Amateurs can only hope to score enough sponsorships and manufacturer support to be able to stay on the road. As an amateur you do get paid what's known as a "contingency" by your bike company, depending on how well you do in a certain race. If you ride a Honda, for example, you can claim a certain amount of money from them if you win a race. The amount awarded per race is determined by the manufacturer, and each one is different. Honda tends to have better contingencies than the other manufacturers.

In pro racing, girls get $600 per moto win from MX Sports. If you win both motos, you get $1,200. Pros also get paid a salary by the manufacturer that sponsors them—but the size of that salary all depends on their contract.

The X Games pay very well—$40,000 for the men's and women's winners. In 2008, the first year women competed in the X

Games, the prize purse was $10,000, then they upped it to $40,000 the following year, in the name of equality.

First Love

I met fellow racer Trey Canard in January of 2006. What can I say . . . he was definitely a cute boy, a cute boy who would become my first boyfriend. Trey is from Elk City, Oklahoma, about five foot seven with reddish hair and pale skin. I was fifteen when we started dating. Trey was always sweet to me—the only times we argued were when our competitive natures clashed. Both of us wanted to win, both of us wanted to be pros, which led to a little friendly competition and ribbing. Whenever my father compared my riding to Trey's, for example, there'd be fireworks. I *hated* that. And for a while in interviews, when anyone asked me what my goals were, I would say, "My goal is to beat Trey Canard."

For me, winning was about identity—it was a way I could express myself and break free of any stereotypes about what it meant to be deaf or be a girl. For Trey, winning was about something else. His father had introduced him to motorcycles, and Trey wanted to make him proud. But before Trey had a chance to make it as a pro, his dad died, on a tractor. The accident happened about two years before we got together. For Trey, winning was about fulfilling his dad's dreams as well as his own. Trey's mom was an inspiration to us all—after Trey's dad died, she didn't miss a beat. She got her son back on the road with a mechanic, and in his rookie year as a pro, 2007, Trey won the national supercross championship. Which tells you a lot about the Canards.

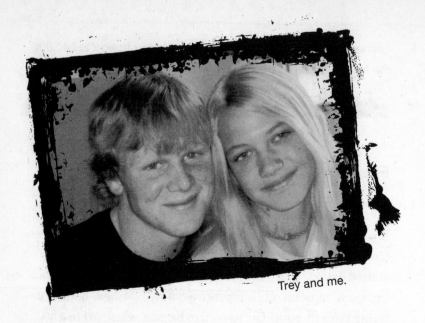
Trey and me.

I remember the first time I actually talked to Trey. He was in Florida training and I happened to be at the same track. A sponsor we both knew introduced us and we got to chatting. He was homeschooled like me, and he loved winning. We exchanged cell numbers and started texting. I taught him how to sign and finger-spell a little so we could communicate more easily. The best thing about being with Trey was that he understood the pressures of being in motocross.

On my sixteenth birthday Trey called up a graphics company to order some vinyl decals for my bike.

"Who are the stickers for?" asked the voice on the phone.

"Ashley Fiolek," said Trey, not even thinking about it.

"Really? Ashley Fiolek? And who is this?" He gave them his information.

"Yeah, nice try. You're not Trey Canard. Hey, I guess you know those two are dating, then?" I guess word had spread of our romance.

We rode together a lot in 2006 and 2007, and I'll admit, I learned a lot. Trey, Ryan Dungey (2009 men's motocross champion), and I were training with the same coach, Shannon Niday, at that time, and working alongside such driven racers pushed me to new levels. After a long day on the dirt, we would go back to our families' respective motor homes, parked at whichever track we were training at, and get cleaned up. At night I might walk over to Trey's motor home and hang out, or he would walk over to ours and hang out with my family. It wasn't like typical teenage dating, where you go to the movies and hold hands. For us, dates revolved around our dirt bikes.

One time, Trey came to Florida to stay with us after breaking his collarbone while testing bikes in California. He was complaining about the pain and as usual, I relished the opportunity to tease him. "Don't be a crybaby," I said, which made him really mad. At the end of the day, I know Trey wanted me to win, and I always wanted him to win. At the same time, I wanted to beat him, but he would never have allowed that to happen. It was the kind of friendly tension that can only push you to be a better rider.

Training Day

In 2006 my dad and I set some pretty tough goals that would require me to work hard—*real hard*. First of all, I wanted to qualify in the boys' 85 cc, age fourteen through fifteen class at Loretta Lynn's. If I did, I knew I'd be one of the first girls to do so. In addition, I also wanted to compete in the women's class, as usual. Which meant I would have to compete in two different sets of qualifiers and regionals for Loretta's.

It was time to get some outside help.

I started working with trainers, who supplemented everything my dad and I were doing. As I mentioned, we spent a couple months with Shannon Niday at his training facility in Texas, alongside Trey and Ryan Dungey. Shannon was an ex–motocross rider himself and had endured several knee surgeries as a result of his injuries on the track. Because of this, he walked with a limp. Shannon is among the best in the field, and what he taught me about getting out of the gate I still use today. It's a secret technique, and maybe I'll tell the world about it in ten years or so. But not just yet.

I also trained with Colleen Millsaps (her son, Davi Millsaps, is my teammate at Honda). She is short like my mom and always wears a visor. She'd drill me and drill me, just like my dad does, and if there was a big jump, she'd say, "You better do it!"

Ronnie Tichenor, one of the fastest supercross riders of the 1980s as well as one of the best coaches in the business, was the one who really started prepping me for life as a pro. Like Shannon, Ronnie also walks with a limp thanks to his dirt bike injuries. His instructions were very technical, and he used a lot of jargon that I couldn't quite get my head around. My parents had to figure out how to sign words like "radius" and "traction" and used a pen and paper to explain them to me diagrammatically. As soon as I could visualize what he was talking about, it all made sense. Once Ronnie realized this, he brought a notepad out with him every time we met.

In June of '06 we visited with Taylor Johnson. Taylor was a really fast amateur but he injured himself a lot and eventually had to drop out of motocross. His dad, Kevin Johnson, had a training center in Pine Mountain, Georgia, where we stayed for a month and a half, working on everything we'd learned with Shannon, Ronnie, and Colleen. Much of our work with the trainers had focused on turns and corners, because that's where kids lose all their time. Jumps—well, you can't really teach someone to jump. You just have to be brave enough to go ahead and do it. You get better by doing it over, again and again. Working with Kevin Johnson at Pine Mountain, I was dirty and muddy for six weeks straight.

May the Best Girl Win

Sarah Whitmore and I had grown very close by this point and were always joking about the day we'd have to race against one another. In truth, she was the one person in the world I didn't want to battle on the track.

"One of these days, you're going to beat me," she would say. I told her no, I would never beat her, and I never would want to pass her. She shook her head.

"Ashley, you're going to beat me—and if anyone's going to beat me, I want it to be you." We decided that on the track, the rule would be "May the best girl win." Off the track, there is no best girl—just best friends.

In 2006 we finally lined up together, at the biggest amateur race of the year, no less—Loretta Lynn's. I had gotten a really good start on my little bike, and we were headed toward a big tabletop jump in the middle of the track. I was in front of Sarah and almost did the jump, but then decided not to at the last minute. Behind me, Sarah had assumed I was jumping. When she realized I wasn't, she hit her brakes and ended up half-jumping, landing hard and ramming right into me.

"I'm sorry! I'm so sorry!"

Of course I had no idea she was saying anything, because I'm deaf. She remembered that a few seconds later and started signing.

"I'M SORRY!"

Sarah was getting sucked up in my back wheel so I turned off the engine and helped disentangle her.

She was about to take off and reenter the race, but I was in trouble—I kept trying to get my bike up but it was stuck in the mud. I couldn't get it to budge. Sarah bent down and helped me pull up my bike while a head honcho at Yamaha, Sarah's sponsor, looked on in horror. He threw his arms up in the air as if to say, "What are you *doing*?" Helping out a rival rider during the biggest race of the year is a major no-no. She came in fourth and I didn't finish—known as a DNF (Did Not Finish) in motocross speak. I just couldn't get my bike to start again.

And there was plenty more drama to come that year at Loretta's. In the second moto of that women's race I passed Jessica Patterson, a WMA champion and the fastest woman in the world, on my little 85 bike. She was riding a 250. People asked me how I had pulled it off and I think it boiled down to sheer hunger. But that was eclipsed by my performance in the boys' fourteen-through-fifteen 85 cc class—forty-one of the best boys in the United States, *and me.* By the time boys reached their mid-teens, they were generally too strong and too fast for girls to be able to keep up. My goal had been to make the top fifteen in the boys' class, and racing against guys like Blake Wharton (now a leading pro), Terren O'Dell, and Lowell Spangler—all the top boys in that age group—I managed to hold my own.

The guys didn't cut me any slack on the track. It was each racer for him- or herself. I hadn't expected or wanted it any different. Boys always tend to race a little rougher than girls, and there was lots of jostling and pushing out of the gate. But I held my own, my eleventh place a significant finish given that everyone was expecting me to crumble under the boys' heat.

Coming in eleventh in the boys' race and overtaking Jessica

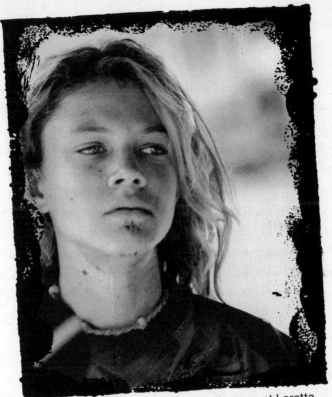

Exhausted and muddy after my many races at Loretta Lynn's, 2006. *Andrew Campo*

Patterson erased all the disappointment surrounding my DNF in the first women's moto—suddenly everyone in the industry was wondering, *Who on earth is this girl?*

Wrench in the Works

A mechanic—or "wrench," as we call them in motocross—is a must for riders like me who are on the road all the time. My dad was still working his job and it had gotten to the point where we needed someone to make sure the bikes were ready to go each race day. As we were expecting I would go pro the next year, a mechanic was a must.

We had met Cody Wolf—everyone calls him C-Wolf—in July of 2006 when I was racing in Ponca City. One of my sponsors made the introduction and mentioned that Cody would be interested in wrenching for me. Sandy-haired and twinkly-eyed, he was only eighteen and still living in Wisconsin with his family. We text-messaged for a couple of months, and eventually my family invited him to come to the Mini Olympics in Florida with us. We spent a whole week together and my parents and I were impressed. My dad and I had talked to other kids his age, and they seemed more wrapped up in partying—but Cody was different. He seemed to understand our program and was a good representative for our family. Most of all, he seemed to enjoy himself too. We asked Cody to come move in with us in Florida, and he accepted. The Fiolek family had grown once again.

A mechanic needs to know how to rip every strip of metal, every bolt, and every piece of plastic off a bike until there's nothing left but a frame. Then he cleans everything and builds it back up to be a complete dirt bike again. That's the only way you can be sure that everything has been inspected, maintained, greased, and lubricated. Cody treated the bike as though it were an extension of his body. He could take a complete engine, split the cases, change my valve assemblies, and inspect my carburetor in his sleep, pretty much.

He set up his workshop at the back of our house in Florida, a twelve-by-fourteen-foot shed that my dad built with a workbench and plenty of room for storage. Like me, Cody is a perfectionist, and motocross is first and foremost. He understood all too well that if he didn't do his job, I could get hurt. But we never had to worry about Cody being under-diligent—in fact we would joke that he had OCD, because he was so organized. His workshop floor was so clean, you could eat off it.

Maintenance Advice

If you're a kid starting out in motocross, there are a few things you should do each time you ride. Check that there's enough gas in the bike and the spokes are tight, and make sure that all your bolts are tightened so nothing's loose or falling off when you're riding. Try to learn how to carry out basic maintenance—whether it's changing oil or changing air filters—and come up with a maintenance time sheet that you can execute yourself. There are lots of little things you can do that will make a world of difference—you just have to put in some effort. When you buy a motorcycle, contact the manufacturer and make sure you get a service manual, which will give you step-by-step advice on how to install, clean, and uninstall parts. Look in your manual to get torque specs—that allows you to set every bolt at its right torque limit so you are not overtightening or leaving things too loose.

A lot of mechanics woo the top amateur boys, because they think that's the surest way into a pro factory team. Cody could have left and worked for some of the top male racers, but he didn't. Instead, he became a part of our family. Now there were five of us in the little motor home, with Cody sleeping in the bunk above the cab. The team had been assembled, and I was ready to go pro.

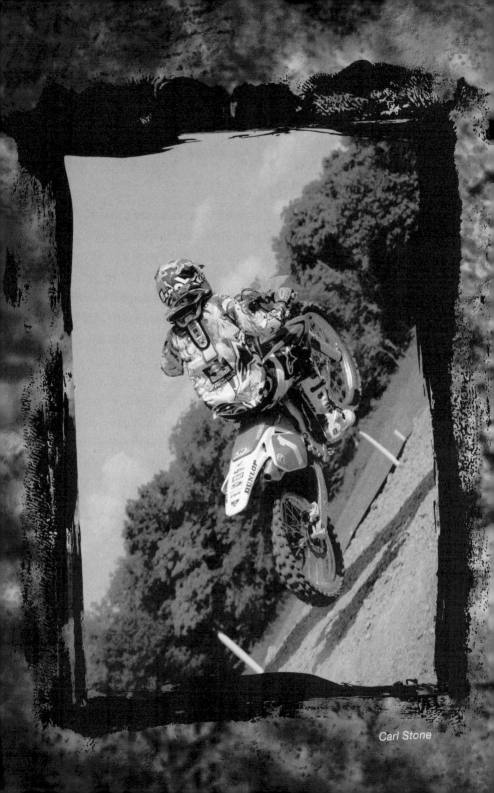

Carl Stone

chapter 6

GOING PRO

Rookie Debut

Miki Keller had been urging me to go pro for a while—under the rules of the WMA, a rider can apply for a professional license as early as her fifteenth birthday. But we waited until I was sixteen before we made the leap. Pro racing presents the motocross racer with a whole new set of challenges. It's faster than amateur racing, it's *gnarlier,* and the tracks are super rough. They've been getting rougher for some years, partially thanks to the popularity of supercross. As interest in supercross has exploded, motocross promoters have started building bigger, supercross-esque jumps outdoors. Bigger jumps equal bigger risk. Suddenly there were doubles and triples where there were none before—and if you come up short on a triple jump, there's a good chance you'll be leaving in an ambulance.

Boys always race their first pro race directly after the last race of the amateur season, Loretta's. We decided that I would race my final Loretta Lynn's in 2007—and then go pro, as planned.

Many in the industry were confused by my decision. "Why don't you want to go back to Loretta's?" asked one promoter. "All the other pro girls do."

"That's the point," I said. "It's got to change."

In the end, I wasn't even able to race Loretta's that year, after breaking my ankle at a qualifier in Ohio. Not being able to say a proper good-bye to Loretta's was heartbreaking, but my excitement at taking part in a real pro race soon perked me up.

The first pro women's race after Loretta's was at Steel City in Pennsylvania, and it was the final race of the season. By the time it came around, the doctors had given me and my ankle the all-clear. Steel City's a tough track—really hard packed, with some good-size jumps. It's especially tough to ride in the rain, as hard-packed tracks tend to be very slippery when wet. Annoyingly, it had been raining for two weeks straight prior, and by the time we arrived for my pro debut, the track was a mud fest. I had won mud races before, but those wins always tended to involve some element of luck. Mud is, after all, the great equalizer.

In my first pro race, I would be lining up against the best female racers in the world—like reigning WMA champion Jessica Patterson, also with Honda. She had dominated the pro series for years, winning the WMA championship in 2000, 2004, 2005, and 2006.

Jessica's known for being reserved, and she generally prefers to keep the competition at a distance. It's not that she's uncomfortable with people—Jessica has a lot of friends. I think she's uncomfortable getting too close to other racers, since she has to compete against them. The guy racers tend to adopt the same attitude—top boys tend not to talk to one another, and they won't be buddies. Jessica and I have talked about what the sport should be like and changes that women need to make. But we don't discuss race strategy or get too friendly. My approach, on the other hand, has always been very people oriented, probably because I'm such a fanatic about communicating. I'll be signing autographs seconds before the two-minute board goes up to start a race. Jessica—or JP, as we call her—needs space to gear up and relax. I tend to toss all my gear out to the fans after a moto—goggles and jerseys, mainly. JP doesn't do that. She's a great rider, but we never really built a friendship—on or off the track. Maybe it was for the best, as she would become my biggest rival.

Barf-a-rama

My pre-race ritual is a somewhat bizarre process that has evolved over years of racing. I always warm up, which means getting on my stationary bike in the motor home, pedaling and working my muscles. Then I go say hello to my dirt bike and double-check my gas. Running out of fuel is the last thing you want to be worrying about on the track.

Then it's time to get dressed—I always put on my left side of gear and boots first. I'll take my helmet and put it on my head—twice. Then I'll check the gas again—three times from the left and three times from the right. For the most part, my ritual has remained the same over the years, right down to the way I put on my helmet, my gloves, and my hair band. It's all about sequencing—I can't start doing one thing until the last is completely finished.

One classic motocross superstition is that if you buy a new helmet, you should toss it onto the ground and scratch it before wearing it. I like to pick up my helmet and kiss it before I put it on. Motocross is a dangerous, gnarly sport and people get hurt on dirt bikes all the time—rituals can help you shift your focus away from the risks.

I always make sure to eat and drink something—although nothing too heavy. Maybe some fruit or toast, and then after practice, I can eat a little more. Again, something light. Directly before a race, some riders will drink a gel pack, a kind of energy supplement that you mix with water for an immediate energy boost. They come in different flavors, like chocolate or banana—and they invariably make me violently ill.

I've been known to throw up on many a starting line, but the gel packs, especially, are a recipe for disaster. I figured this out in the spring of 2008 at a track called Oak Hill during the GNC championship. The GNC is primarily an amateur race but they had a pro class that I wanted to race as a warm-up for my pro debut.

I was already in bad shape, recovering from an accident the week before in which a male racer on a practice track had landed his bike directly on top of me. I spent one night in the hospital and took it easy the whole week, hoping to recover in time for the GNC. Bruised and broken, I made it to the racetrack, and shortly before my first moto, I tried a gel pack for the first time. My stomach churned, and its contents projectiled onto the mud. I didn't stop throwing up until seconds before the gate dropped. Somehow, I ended up winning the moto—but my victory was short-lived. JP protested me for passing her on a yellow flag, which is against the rules, and they took away the championship. I conceded defeat, and vowed never again to go near a gel pack. Yuck!

The most important part of my ritual is prayer. Before each race, my family and I will sign a prayer each, usually with me starting and then my parents following. Prayer is such a big part of our lives, not just in motocross, but every day. Before a race, however, our prayers take on added poignancy.

"Dear God, please help me do my best and keep me safe. And above all, help me to have fun. I know that You have a plan for me, God. I have done all the work I can do, and the rest I am leaving up to You."

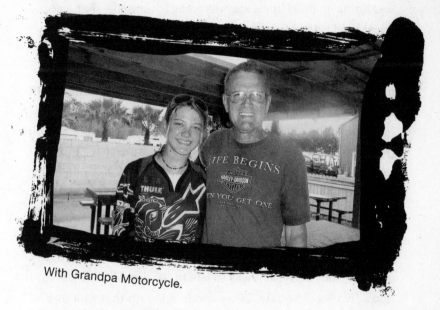

With Grandpa Motorcycle.

There's something calming about leaving things up to God. On the starting line, just before the gate drops, I say another prayer (in my head), cross myself, and look up. Finally, I'm ready to go.

Mud Bath

As I was getting into position at Steel City, I spotted Grandpa Motorcycle standing by a fence lining the track. Earlier that day, he had let me bleach a number 67 in the hair on the back of his head. All motocross riders are given a number when they start racing, and mine was 67. You're supposed to keep it for the entirety of your career. I was also wearing a new neck brace with a sticker on the back that said PRO, given to me by our friend Geoff Patterson from the Leatt brace company. That sticker is still on our refrigerator today.

Our first moto was early, at nine thirty A.M. Sarah Whitmore was lining up and I knew she was going to do well—she's a confident mud rider. Meanwhile Jessica Patterson was points away from winning the women's championship for a fifth time. I got a good start and found myself neck-and-neck with Sarah Whitmore for the holeshot. Sarah won it by a hair's breadth—then ended up zooming ahead of me. Vanessa Florentino, a talented racer from New Mexico, overtook me next, and I hung on in third for as long as I could. But I kept falling in the deep mud. By the second lap, Sarah was way ahead of everyone and ended up winning the moto. I came in sixth.

We had to wait until the very end of the day to race our second moto. I was on the line and raring to go when we were informed that our second moto was going to be cut by five minutes, probably because it was so late in the day. My dad was furious. "No way," he said. "They would *never* do that to a men's moto, unless it was pouring with rain or there was a lightning storm." He was angry that our racing was deemed less important than the men's, despite all the hard work and dedication that we'd put into it. The race administrators reluctantly agreed to keep the race at its original length.

The gate dropped and this time, I got the holeshot—not easy, as the opening stretch was up a hill and I was riding a 125, in contrast to the other girls' 250s. Luckily, the weather conditions had improved and the track wasn't as muddy as before. I was in first place for a few laps with Jessica Patterson hot on my heels. She passed me in the double-jumps section at the top of the track, and Sarah came up behind me too. Nerves must have gotten the better of me, because I crashed off a tabletop jump, riding in way too high a gear. I got on the bike again straightaway and finished the second moto in third place. It wasn't my best performance.

"You were hitting the rear brake too late into the corners," my dad pointed out afterward. "And why were you sitting down so early?" I couldn't argue—he wasn't saying anything that wasn't true. Nonetheless a holeshot award and a third-place moto finish wasn't too shabby for my first day as a pro. Jessica Patterson won the championship a fifth time, with Tarah Gieger in second place, E-Bash in fourth, and Sarah sixth in the overall rankings. The race reports said I had put in a "solid rookie ride"; I felt proud of myself.

Trey sent me a text message after the race. "How are ya? Nice race!" I smiled. I knew he was around, on the track, but I had no idea where. Probably hanging with his buddies.

In a year together, we had only been able to see each other ten times, mainly at races, and a couple times when he came to visit me in Florida, and I went to see him in Oklahoma. We had so much in common—our drive, our love for the sport—but motocross is a tough industry for relationships, we learned.

The busier and more successful we became, the less available we were to one another. I know we were both pretty young, still teenagers, but we were both fully committed to our careers. Eventually the mud seeped into our relationship and with so little time spent together, we decided it would be better if we just remained friends. Detaching was hard at first, as I had grown close to him. He was my first boyfriend, after all. But now, it seemed like things were cool between us.

"Thanks!" I texted back. "See you soon!"

All Grown Up

Once the dust had settled and the family returned to St. Augustine, I took a big step. I bought my very first truck, a Ford F150 in burgundy. I figured it was about time I had my own set of wheels, wheels that I could take to Wendy's or to the mall, not just make jumps with. With the winnings I'd been making, I was able to pay cash.

"Why don't you let me buy you a truck too?" I signed to my dad in the showroom. "You spent all your money helping me race dirt bikes—it's the least I could do."

He wouldn't let me, insisting he was perfectly happy with his 1998 Nissan. That's the thing—my parents have never been in it for the money. As strongly as they believe that I and all other women should be properly paid for the skill and risk level involved in racing a dirt bike, they've always been very hands-off when it comes to my winnings. My dad has been involved in training me for years, and my mom has been in charge of all travel arrangements and working on interviews—but it's something they do for the love of it. They've never taken a dime. They don't even charge me a management fee, unlike many parents in the sport.

Tooling around St. Augustine in my new truck, I realized something—I actually don't like to drive. In fact, I generally prefer it if someone else drives me. I spend so much time navigating dirt that roads and traffic feel somewhat alien.

So aside from the truck, what was I going to treat myself with? Growing up racing a dirt bike, I've never really had much desire for anything too flashy. I don't need a big TV or gadgets, and I'm not one for buying clothes—I get all mine for free—so when I do have a little money I generally spend it all on food. If I could go out to eat every day, three times a day, I would. Sushi is my absolute favorite. P. F. Chang's for Chinese. Wendy's is my favorite for fast food. Oh, and steak—I love Outback Steakhouse. *Yum.*

E-Bashed

I never worry too much about being injured; focusing on the worst-case scenario is a real distraction. Plus, I always just assume that God has a plan for me, so what happens is what's meant to happen. But when my *friends* get hurt—that's a different story. That's when I start to understand how my parents must feel.

In February 2008, E-Bash went down hard at Lake Whitney Motocross Park in Texas and was airlifted to JPS Hospital in Fort Worth with a torn-up spleen, a broken pelvis, and damage to her pancreas. She was bleeding internally and even though she's a tough gal, it sounded like she was pretty beat-up. I was home in Florida when it happened. I knew deep down she would be OK, but still, it took nearly three weeks before she was well enough to leave the hospital. She was on an IV drip and a cyst had formed over the torn-up part of her pancreas. I've never really suffered internal injuries like that—just good, clean broken bones for me. So she was constantly in my prayers.

A Woman in the World

Now that I had gone pro, we'd been approached with a few offers of management and we ended up signing with Hardcard Holdings, a sports agency, for representation. Honda, Oakley, Alpinestars, and Red Bull were already my sponsors, and in April I signed with Vans, the shoe company, making me the first girl to join the Vans Motocross family. Vans boys included Ryan Villopoto, one of the top men. Today, my key sponsors are American Honda, Red Bull, Alpinestars, T-Mobile, Smith, Leatt, and Robb Beams, a personal trainer and nutritionist, whose company MotoEndurance creates tailor-made training and nutrition programs for many pro motocrossers.

I was also gearing up for my first trip to Europe, where I'd be competing in a few rounds of the prestigious FIM World Motocross series. I couldn't wait!

My dad and I left Florida on Wednesday, May 7, 2008. Destination: Gorna Rositsa, Bulgaria, where the Grand Prix of Bulgaria (the first race of the FIM World Motocross series) was being held. Our first stop was Italy—it was already breakfast time there when we landed, but no time for morning gelato. We only had a few minutes to make our connecting flight to Bulgaria, so my dad and I raced from the plane to the baggage claim to get our bags.

We usually travel light, but this time we had packed some parts that I specifically needed for this race. When we showed up at the baggage claim, our bags started coming out straightaway, before anyone else's. The first one came out, then the next one, then the next—I looked at my dad and we were both surprised at how fast our luggage was showing up. Then we realized something was missing—my bike suspension. We continued to wait until the belt stopped. *Nothing.* Had my suspension fallen out of the plane over the ocean? I was feeling pretty nervous by now.

My dad went over to customer service and asked what was going on. I normally keep my suspension in a gun case, which I know is a little unusual, but that's how I make sure it stays protected. The gun case had freaked out a few people, apparently, and the airport folks were inspecting it very carefully. After establishing that there were no weapons in my gun case, they said they would be happy to send it on to the Czech Republic for us. *But the*

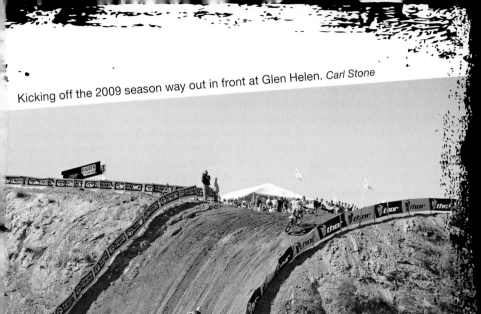

Kicking off the 2009 season way out in front at Glen Helen. *Carl Stone*

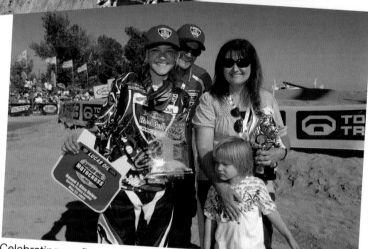

Celebrating my first win of the 2009 season with my family. *Carl Stone*

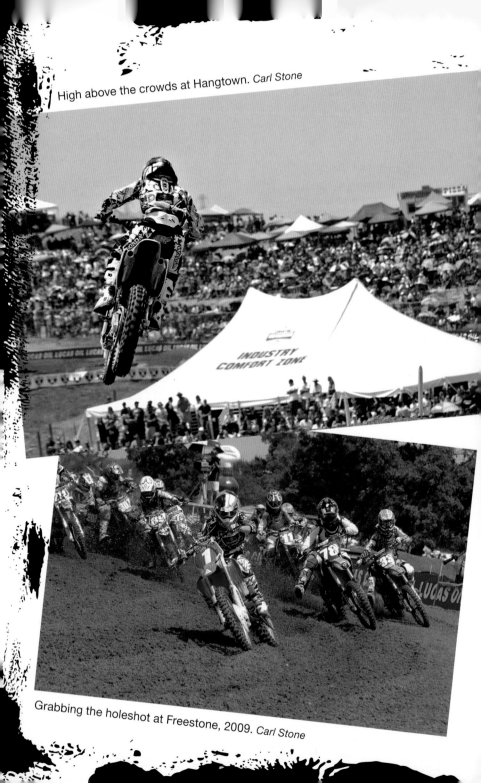

High above the crowds at Hangtown. *Carl Stone*

Grabbing the holeshot at Freestone, 2009. *Carl Stone*

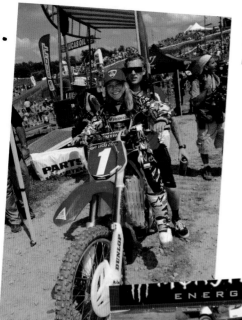

With my mechanic, C-Wolf before the start of the 2009 race at High Point. *Carl Stone*

Lined up at the High Point starting line. *Carl Stone*

My dad translates my podium speech for me at High Point. *Carl Stone*

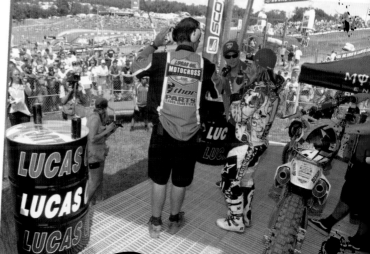

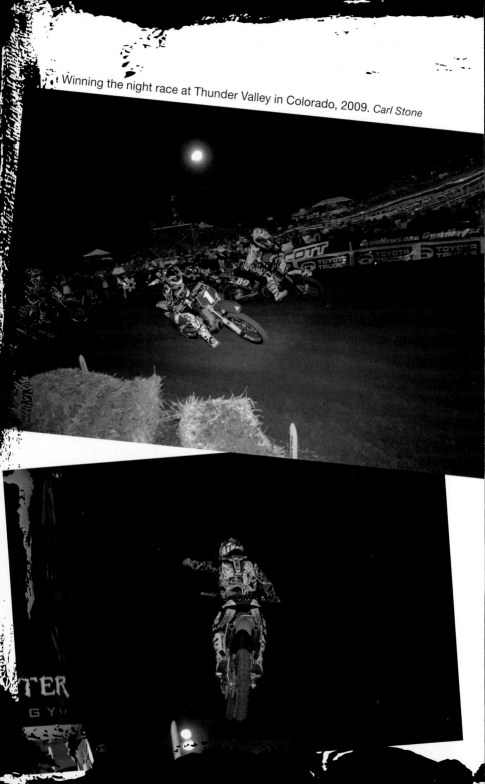

Winning the night race at Thunder Valley in Colorado, 2009. *Carl Stone*

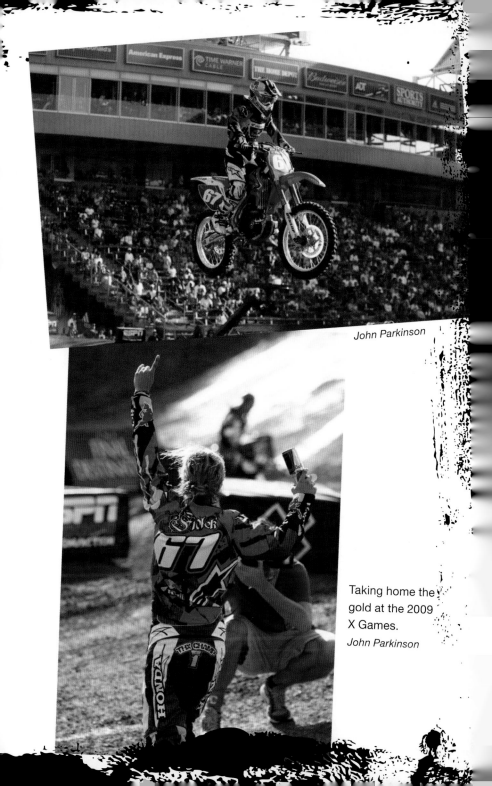

John Parkinson

Taking home the gold at the 2009 X Games.

John Parkinson

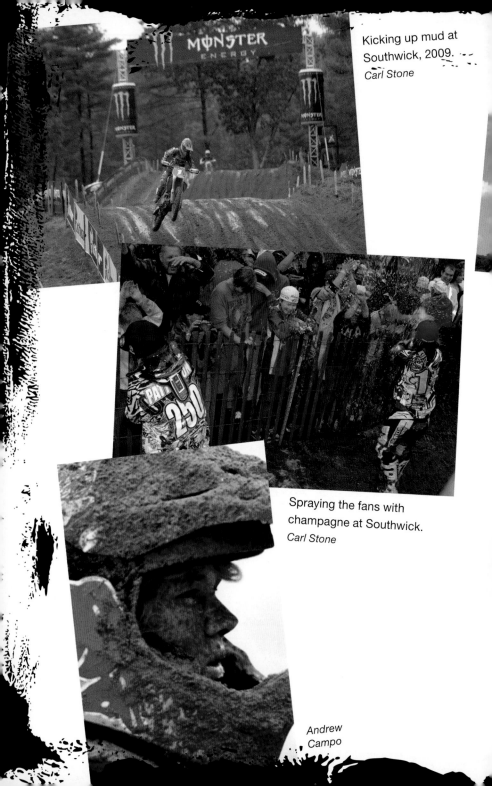

Kicking up mud at
Southwick, 2009.
Carl Stone

Spraying the fans with
champagne at Southwick.
Carl Stone

*Andrew
Campo*

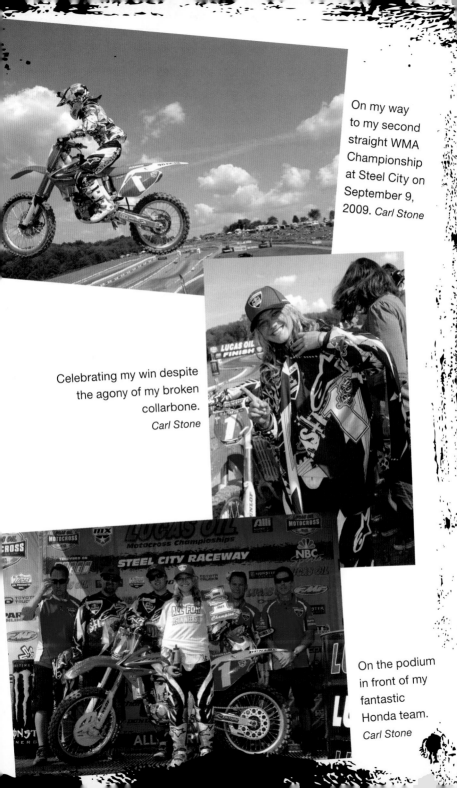

On my way to my second straight WMA Championship at Steel City on September 9, 2009. *Carl Stone*

Celebrating my win despite the agony of my broken collarbone. *Carl Stone*

On the podium in front of my fantastic Honda team. *Carl Stone*

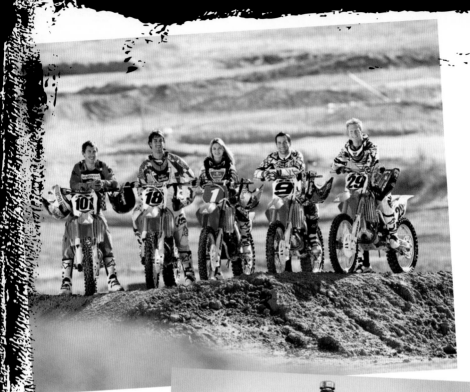

Team Honda, 2009.
Courtesy of American Honda

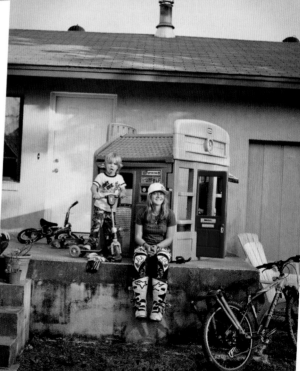

Hanging out at home with my little brother, Kicker, the next generation of Fiolek motocrosser.

race was in Bulgaria, not the Czech Republic! Luckily, just before my dad blew his top, an airport worker came over and said they had found my suspension and were putting it on the right flight. It was a lucky escape, and I was hoping it wasn't a bad omen. I was excited about this trip and didn't want anything to ruin it.

We landed in Sofia, the capital of Bulgaria, and commenced our drive to the track, situated just outside the thousand-year-old town of Sevlievo, in the north. Sevlievo was a good 110 miles from the airport and we were following another driver to get there. That drive might have been the most stressful part of the whole entire trip. The roads were extremely narrow, crowded with work vehicles, transports, and people crossing with little warning. When the driver we were following passed a vehicle, my dad had to pass it too. As our car didn't have great pickup, we had a few near misses—in fact, a couple of times I thought we were toast. But my dad always darted away from the oncoming traffic at the last second.

We arrived in Sevlievo three hours later, exhausted, and checked into our hotel. Our room overlooked the Gorna Rositsa racetrack and it was majestic—built in 1959, it had been reconstructed in 2000 and turned into a top motocross facility, one of the best in the world (it won the 2006 and 2007 Best Organizer Awards in the FIM Off Road Awards). It's shaped like an amphitheater, so the spectators have a great view of what's going on. And boy, do they love their motocross in Bulgaria—in fact, the Bulgarian Grand Prix is one of the most important events in the country's sporting calendar. With that on my mind, and after more than twenty-four hours of travel, we hit the hay.

The next morning was the women racers' first practice, and that's when I noticed how differently the Europeans did things. We were allowed three full half hours to practice on the track—

enough time to stop and talk to your mechanic, make adjust-
ments to wheel pressure, and fine-tune the bike to the course.
In the States, girls don't get that kind of time. The track was
challenging, not a lot of double or triple jumps but up-and-down
hills with a variety of turns. I would be racing against some of
the best girls in the world today—including Livia Lancelot from
France, the number one racer in the world—and I was the only
American girl racing. I finished fourth in the timed qualifier, the
top five girls all within a half second of each other. I knew it was
going to be a great race.

Eleven A.M. the following day was when the real fun began—
our first moto. In a grand prix race, the motos are longer, twenty
minutes plus two laps, whereas in America national races are
fifteen minutes plus one lap. The crowd was smaller than at
American races—maybe two thousand people or so, mostly
Bulgarians—but what they lacked in numbers they made up

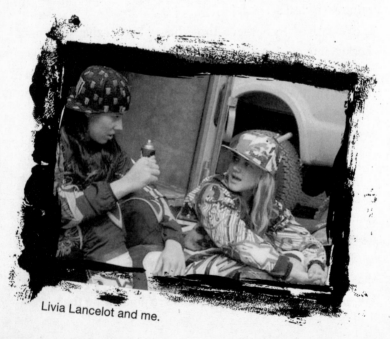

Livia Lancelot and me.

for in passion. In Europe, the tracks aren't groomed or fixed up in between practices and the race itself. In America, riders will yell for the tractors to hit the tracks whenever they can, saying they need tidier tracks because they are traveling at such high speeds. The time it takes to groom the track is normally shaved off women's races.

Under FIM rules, only the rider is allowed at the gate, so I had to set up my own trench and starting blocks. My dad normally does that for me, and it's heavy work—but I figured it out OK. I had a great gate pick and got a good start, running the pace of the leaders—then I stalled my motor. Luckily, I was on the downslope of a hill, so I was able to restart it and only lost a few seconds. Maria Franke, a German rider, was my closest competitor for that race—we passed each other four times. I ended up finishing third, thrilled to have competed in my very first European grand prix.

The second moto was a little more hair-raising. It had started raining and the track became super slick. Riders were sliding everywhere—it felt like surfing a mudslide. I got in a good jump, and just after the first turn I made a pass for the lead—but that didn't last too long. The European girls were hauling in a major way, and I ended up falling behind a little. I was jumping toward the finish line when Larissa Papenmeier came in a little too close and we ended up hitting each other. *Bam!* That familiar dizzy feeling and the shock in my lungs as we went down hard. I prayed to God—*Please help me get out of this.*

Somehow, I pulled myself up with the bike still running and took off again but got stuck behind some lappers. I was all the way back in tenth place and it took all the strength I had left to make it across the finish line. Livia won, and I came in third place overall on points—can you believe that after all that, I made the podium?

And what a podium it was—in Bulgaria, and in FIM races generally, the women's podium doesn't feel like an afterthought. The top three girls were allowed to have their bikes up with them and we gave press conferences after each and every round, just like the men. Back home, promoters generally treat women, even pros, as though they're not really part of the program. Girls often don't get to park in the same area as boys, we get shorter motos, and until recently, we were rarely invited to press conferences. In Bulgaria, the respect people had for female racers was obvious. That experience flipped a switch inside me. I realized *this* was how it was supposed to be.

Sacred Turf

Spring rolled around and it was time for the 2008 WMA championship to start. This time, my eye was on the prize. I'd be racing on sacred turf, on some of the oldest and most challenging racetracks in America in a series of six races. (The men run twelve races per season, but that's because they have greater financial support; most pro girls simply wouldn't be able to afford to travel to twelve races each season.)

Each track has a personality, a history, and a set of challenges all its own—that's part of what makes the pro championship so fun. Riders have to adapt to the different tracks and their little quirks. Most of them take only a few minutes to lap, but one might be clay, one might be sand, and one might be hard packed. The layouts vary from track to track, too—some have more jumps, and some are more wide open and fast.

Hangtown in Sacramento is a loamy, rocky track with steep jumps more in the style of supercross, the kind that shoot you up way high in the air. When jumps are that steep you have to be precise with your landing position—falling out of the sky, your hope is to land right on the down side of the next jump, which helps absorb the impact.

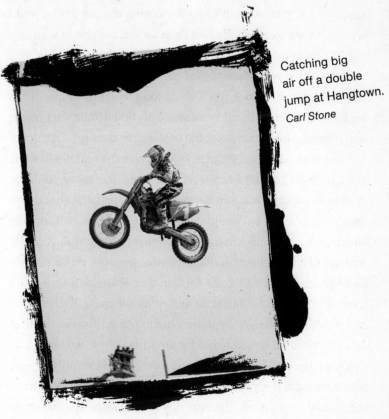

Catching big air off a double jump at Hangtown.
Carl Stone

At Thunder Valley in Lakewood, Colorado, races run at night, and the altitude can make engines lose their power. Southwick in Massachusetts is a deep sand track and really rough—the going is often slowest at Southwick, and the sand can get in the engines and cause mechanical problems as the day goes on.

And Away She Goes

Hangtown, at the end of May 2008, was my first pro race of the season. I was determined to make an impression—this time, unlike at Steel City, I was actually competing to win a title. I had received a fair amount of press for joining the pro ranks, and I wanted to show everybody that I was indeed capable of winning; not just races—but championships.

Hangtown was also memorable because of the sheer *chaos* that led up to it. It took us twice as long to get to California as we had anticipated, thanks to a series of stalled flights, blunders, and missed connections. Not the best way to start my first series. We had booked a hotel room in Jacksonville the night before our six A.M. flight to Sacramento (via Atlanta), just so we could be sure to be on time. But just because *we* were on time, that didn't mean our *plane* was. The plane left the tarmac at Jacksonville so late, we ended up missing our connecting flight in Atlanta. Instead of flying direct to Sacramento, we were rerouted into San Francisco via Salt Lake City. In San Francisco, we rented a car and sped to Sacramento as fast as we could. Kicker, who had never flown before, kept announcing that this was the first and last time he would travel by airplane. When we landed in Oakland, the airline staff informed us they had lost my luggage, which contained my riding gear. By this point, I didn't even have the energy to get mad. The next day Kicker woke up, turned to my dad, and said, "Papa, that was the worst day of my life."

Then, adding insult to injury, we arrived to a completely inadequate setup for us girls at Hangtown. While the boys could park their bikes and set up base camp close to the track, the girls were told to set up way, way far from the track. I remember my poor mom having to push Kicker up and down the rock face in his stroller, like a mountain goat. Having just gotten back from Europe, where we had received the red-carpet treatment, I was distinctly unimpressed. It seemed ridiculous—and insulting—that the women pros weren't allowed to park with the men professionals. (In 2009 the parking situation would be different; women would park in the paddock area. Maybe someone said something—I like to imagine it was my dad, with steam coming out of his ears.)

Our prayers before my first pro race of my first pro season race were the same as they always were. We weren't looking for any kind of magic; I had already done my homework. Now the rest was up to God.

Jessica Patterson dashed straight out of the gate in the first moto, taking the holeshot as if to say "Look who's boss." I was right behind her, speeding round the first turn. Then at the second turn, *bang*—I accidentally slipped into neutral and crashed. I watched Sarah Whitmore and most of the other girls make their way around me.

Um, could this be *any worse?* I thought.

I was on the ground for just fifteen seconds or so before jumping back on the bike. By this point I was in second to last place—nearly the whole field had passed me by. *Stay focused,* I told myself, and got to work eating up the gap. I kept charging, kept passing, and suddenly there were only four girls ahead of me. Jessica fell, as did two other girls, and before I knew it, Sarah and I were battling for the lead. On the fifth lap, I pulled ahead of my friend—all's fair in love and motocross—and prayed I could keep my hold on the lead. I kept thinking about what Sarah had said to me—*"One day you're going to beat me"*—and I knew that she would want me to race my best. The crowd was going nuts—I could see people jumping up and down and waving; they couldn't believe I had pulled forward from last to first place.

The remaining three laps of the eight-lap moto were among the longest in my life. And when I crossed the finish line I wasn't even sure I had won . . . until I saw Rick Wernli, our dear friend and occasional mechanic, on the sidelines holding up a pit board that said YOU WON! I couldn't believe it; I had taken the first moto of the season. Jessica, the reigning champion, had come in eighth. I had grown accustomed to keeping my emotions under control, especially when it came to big celebrations—but this time, I let myself really feel the excitement in my heart. What an auspicious start.

The next day, there was no way I *wasn't* going to get the holeshot. Starts are my specialty, and I'd let myself down the previous moto. Out the gate I took the holeshot, but Jessica was hot on my heels. On the second lap, I tried to make a jump and landed badly, getting a face full of dirt. Jessica sped away ahead of me, as did Tarah Gieger, then SoCal rider Tatum Sik. I pulled myself together, well aware I had a battle ahead of me. I managed to make it back up to finish in third. The final results were 1-3 (first in the first moto, third in the second moto) for me and 8-1 (eighth in the first moto, first in the second) for Jessica. Jessica had won the second moto—but I won Hangtown overall, on points, thanks to her poor eighth-place finish in the first moto. I had beaten the top women riders in the world in my first race of the 2008 pro season. Ladies and gentlemen, I was officially a contender.

The Motocross Points System

In pro motocross, championships are won based on the total number of points a rider accumulates over the season. You win championship points for each race according to your official finishing position, with points being awarded all the way up to twentieth place per moto. Come in first, and you win 25 points. Second place gets you 22 points, third place 20 points and so on. Twentieth position bags you just one point. If there's ever a tie for the championship, the winner is determined based on the number of races won during the series.

Now what if there's a points tie in an individual race? Well, races are made up of two motos, and the second moto is always given more weight, the reasoning being that fatigue and track deterioration will make the second moto tougher than the first. For example—let's say you win the first moto of a race (25 points), but come second in the second moto (22 points), and you're tied on points with another rider who came second in the first moto (22 points), but won the second moto (25 points). Even though you both scored the same number of points, the race will go to the other rider, because the second moto win is worth more. It's a little confusing at first, but the system works, and it's easy to understand once you get the hang of it.

Of course, I was happy to have won my first pro overall, but my dad had some stern words for me. We had a rule—if I got first place but wasn't riding to the best of my ability, he would tell me. And if I came in last and had done everything I was supposed to do, then he would congratulate me. In this race, he felt that I could have easily avoided coming off the bike in the second moto. Plus I had been reluctant to take a double jump, even though it was small. He noticed I wasn't jumping it because my corner speed was too slow. Jessica did jump it, and then when I tried too, I did so halfheartedly, and that was why I crashed. My eagle-eyed dad never missed a beat—he saw how my hesitation had cost me the moto. Even though I knew he was just trying to do his job as my coach, it was definitely one of those days when I just wished he could have been happier for me, as a dad.

Then we got some news that everyone could be excited about—Miki had worked her magic, and women's motocross had finally been accepted into the X Games. Women BMXers and skaters had already been competing in the X Games for some time, so this was way overdue. The ten top women in motocross would compete for gold at the games, which were taking place in Los Angeles that July. Best of all, I was among the honored few who had been asked to participate. We didn't have too much time to celebrate though; I had to get myself into fighting form for the next race of the women's championship—at Freestone County Raceway in Texas.

Bat out of Hell

It was the first week of June in Wortham, Texas, and the heat was overwhelming. Even the boys were dropping like flies—some riders had fallen off their bikes and passed out from heat exhaustion in the middle of their motos. Luckily, I was used to extreme temperatures. Enduring the icy winters of Michigan and then Florida's humid summers had made me immune to any kind of weather. Even so, that day I could have used an ice pop.

I was still feeling confident after my win the previous week. So for the first moto, I busted out of the gates and took the holeshot. Again, Jessica Patterson was nudging my tail. For the whole race we battled it out like two gladiators in chariots, neck and neck. She just wouldn't let up. The adrenaline was pumping through my veins, and combined with the insane heat I thought I might melt under my gear and helmet. But keeping cool—psychologically, at least—was the name of the game. Any mistake, just one error of judgment, would cost me the race.

I could see the finish line in the distance and kept my mind steely, my thoughts focused. As we neared, I could feel the energy of her bike next to me. I had to work really hard to pull away from Jessica. I started to edge away . . . inch by inch I could feel myself stretching farther away from her and I crossed the finish line half a bike length ahead of her. I threw up on the track afterward, frazzled and unaware that the media was describing our race as "one of the greatest battles of women's motocross history."

The second Texas moto rolled around the following day. Tensions *and* temperatures continued to ride high. There were way more people crowding the sidelines to watch us women race this time. Which is what I'm all about—bringing more people to women's racing, entertaining and thrilling them as much as the boys!

I grabbed another holeshot with Jessica right behind me and resumed battle, kicking up a cloud of Texas dust. I was enjoying the rivalry that was evolving between us. It was testing all the things I had worked on with my dad—not just technique, but mental resolve and determination. I felt calm and confident. As we came into a corner together, Jessica lost her grip and stalled her bike. I cruised across the finish line about ten minutes later, forty-five seconds ahead of the rest of the field.

On the podium, race officials handed me a bottle of champagne. I had no idea what I was supposed to do with it. I looked to Sarah as if to say "Now what?" She was laughing, as were the other girls. Sarah motioned to me to shake the bottle. *Oh . . . I get it! I'm supposed to spray this all over everyone!* I made sure I got Sarah good. Then she started pouring champagne on me too. It was a refreshing way to cool down after a race.

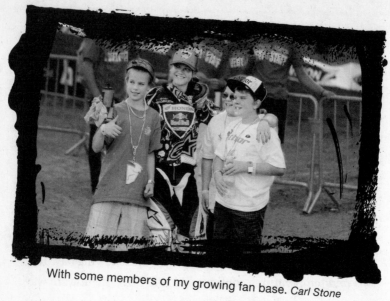

With some members of my growing fan base. *Carl Stone*

I was supposed to go back to Europe to race in Germany, but because I'd won the last two WMA races, the American promoters asked me to stay. They wanted to make sure I wouldn't miss the third race of the WMA season at Thunder Valley, in Lakewood, Colorado. The fans, apparently, were excited to see how this rivalry between me and Jessica would unfold.

Thundering On

Before we committed to staying though, we had a couple of requests. The women were being offered a terrible slot in the Thunder Valley schedule, with no TV time. So we told the promoter that I was not going to cancel my trip to Europe unless we were offered the coverage we deserved. Now that I was doing so well, I had a little bit of leverage and I intended to use it. I'm not sure if it had anything to do with what we said, but the race was moved around to a time slot that made sense, and we decided to stay.

Thunder Valley is a picturesque, mountainous track with pine trees dotting it here and there and expansive views of the Denver skyline. Its altitude robs our engines of power and riders always have to adjust their jetting—the system that sends fuel to the engine—when racing there. The races there are run at night, giving the event a cool, mystical feel.

Moto one, I sped out of the gate and scored the holeshot. This time Tarah Gieger was the one behind me, trying to edge me out of the way. It was all I could do to stay ahead of her. We traded first and second positions all the way to the last lap, until I passed Tarah and managed to hold on. *I could get used to all this winning,* I thought. In the second moto, I didn't get such a good start, but I kept my head throughout and won Thunder Valley on points, again. I could not have been more thrilled with my season so far!

Race number four took place right at the end of July, at Washougal MX Park up in Washington State. It's a pretty track—the surroundings are woody and the track is mainly clay, which means it's a little more hard packed and traction is limited. There aren't many jumps, but it's very, very fast, which is heaven for people like Jessica, Tarah, and me.

I knew I had to ride a little cautiously at Washougal, having broken my wrist just ten days beforehand while training for the X Games at the Red Bull compound in California. My left wrist had been encased in a custom-made hot-pink brace, designed to keep my bones in place. And while it was still broken, some serious rehab involving a cold laser and bone stimulator ensured it wasn't as painful as before.

I won the first moto, with Jessica right there behind me, and I came in second in the second moto, with Jessica in first place. Second motos always count for more in motocross, so this time, Jessica got to win overall. But the championship was far from over.

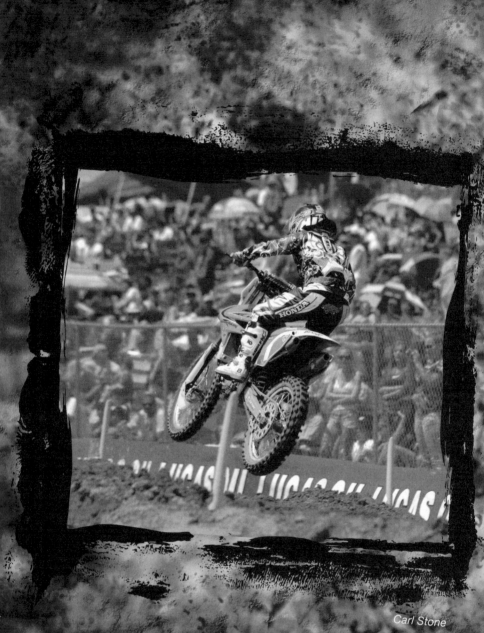

Carl Stone

chapter 7

HURRY UP AND HEAL

It was July 30, 2008, the morning before the fourteenth annual X Games kicked off. For the first time in the games' history, women motocrossers would be allowed to compete. Miki had been working toward this for years—there was simply no bigger event in the action sports calendar than the X Games. Now millions of sports fans around the planet would be watching women dirt bikers on network TV. If ever there was a chance to bring our sport to a wider audience, this was it.

We knew the X Games was going to be a race unlike any other—for starters, it was taking place on one of the toughest, most gnarly supercross tracks in the world, in the Home Depot Center in Carson, California. In that sense, calling it a "motocross" event was something of a misnomer—this wasn't going to be *anything* like the wide-open rural racing we were used to. The X Games is an indoor event, for starters. Walking onto the track at the Home Depot Center, I wondered if this was how gladiators felt before they were fed to the lions—it was the most daunting track I had ever seen. No women in the WMA had substantial experience riding a supercross track as hard packed and triple infested as this one. The finish-line jump alone—a suicidal metal ramp that propelled racers seventy-five feet in the air—was enough to make me question our sanity.

"Not sure my bike will survive!" a fellow racer had texted me earlier that day, echoing a sentiment that many of the girls had already expressed. Most of us had scrambled to replace the suspension on our bikes, because we knew they were about to get majorly pummeled. Our suspension companies seemed overly casual about it all. They didn't seem to grasp what we were about to put our bikes—and our bodies—through.

"Supercross suspension? *For the girls?* OK . . ."

Ten of us had been invited to participate, and the X Games, we learned, is heavily focused on entertainment. The tracks are built with maximum viewer satisfaction in mind. Although we were never expressly told as much, it was understood that our participation was very much a "trial" for us. Collectively, we had to prove to the X Games committee that women motocrossers were just as exciting to watch as the men. In that sense, we were in it as a team.

Bruised Earth

With less than twenty-four hours to go before my X Games debut, Mom, Dad, Kicker, and I found ourselves in the sleepy mountain ranges that surround Lake Piru in Southern California. We were headed for the Red Bull compound, a private thousand-acre off-roading paradise and elite motorsports training facility, where I had been preparing for the X Games all month. Less formal than an academy, more exclusive than a country club, it was a hotbed of motocross, supercross, and freestyle activity.

The compound is in the middle of nowhere. "What's the address?" my mom had asked Red Bull the first time we visited.

"Oh, there isn't an actual address," said the voice on the other end of the line. The road the training facility sits on didn't even have a name, apparently. "Just drive through the little town and pass by the cattle farms and the shooting range and you'll come to a cow crossing. Go over it, head down the sandy road until you pass another cattle ranch and then some stables, and then go around the bend. You'll see it."

There was no cell phone reception where we were headed—just some of the most beautiful, rugged California scenery imaginable: glimmering yellow hillsides crisscrossed with weaving dirt roads, and mountain vistas that seemed to go on forever. Below us lay the compound—we saw its supercross track, motocross track, and ramps for freestyle riders.

I got to work, practicing jumps on the supercross track. In the back of my head, as I'm sure was the case with a few other girls, was a nagging thought: *Is it really worth risking my safety for one shot at winning the X Games when I've still got the rest of the WMA championship to finish?* I tried to push that concern from my mind. This was the first year girls had been allowed to race motocross at the X Games—I should have felt honored, not apprehensive.

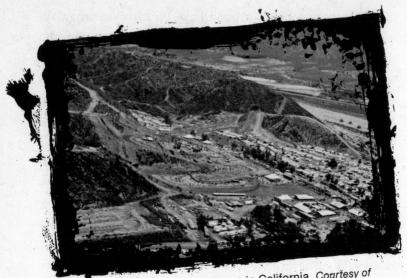

Glen Helen motocross raceway in California. *Courtesy of Glen Helen Raceway*

Unlike a motocross track, which allows for a certain sense of freedom, supercross tracks can feel like a minefield. Each turn brings some new hazard—back-to-back jumps, whoops, and other obstacles—all of which make for a thrilling show and certainly a few broken bones. I wanted to make sure I was ready for an especially gnarly triple jump in the X Games course and accelerated into a similar-looking triple on the practice track. The results were catastrophic—I soared into the air with such speed that I flipped, came off the bike, and plummeted back to the earth, landing on my head.

Blood stained the earth, turning it a muddy burgundy. I was crying and screaming, which wasn't like me. My mom and dad raced over to where I was lying. "Don't move, Ashley, just don't move," my mom signed, and my dad had to gently hold me down to prevent me from squirming. We were all too aware of the angle at which I had landed—if I had damaged my neck or spine, one false move could result in paralysis. My parents carefully removed my neck brace. It was broken in two places—had I not been wearing it I probably would have broken my neck. They carried me inside to the medical area and slowly peeled off my gear. My back was covered in contusions and was so badly scraped, my mom later commented that it looked "like chopped liver." (Which happens to be one of my least favorite foods.)

My left side was especially torn up, and I could barely move my left arm—as we feared, my wrist was in bad shape again. A sports doctor put my left arm in a sling. "You're going to be OK," my mom signed to me, a look of relief on her face. I was grateful that my injuries were relatively superficial, but I couldn't conceal my disappointment. The X Games were tomorrow, and there was no way I was going to be able to race in this condition.

Later we found out that many of the girls' suspension companies had assumed we would be racing on a pared-down supercross track, rather than the same extreme track that the supercross boys usually raced on. The track claimed its victims the following day—one of my fellow girl racers, Alisa Nix, broke both wrists coming down off the seventy-five-foot metal finish ramp and she never fully recovered. The following year, our suspension companies vowed they would step up their game—but for me it was too late.

Part of me just wanted to crawl under a rock and hide. But I knew I'd kick myself if I missed this historic event entirely. We drove to the stadium, and my mom helped me to the bleachers. Limping through the hordes of extreme-sports fans, I was heartened by how excited the young crowd seemed to watch my sport. Sitting in the sidelines, chewing weakly on a pretzel, I watched as my friend Tarah Gieger rode up a storm, taking home gold in the first X Games women's motocross competition. On the Jumbotron screens she waved in excitement, and I realized this was a victory for all of us.

Tactical Riding

I had three weeks to heal in between the X Games and the fifth WMA series race, at the MX338 racetrack in Southwick, Massachusetts. Nestled in the Pioneer Valley with the Congamond Lakes on the south side and Sodom Mountain in the west, the track lies in an outstandingly beautiful part of the country. Its beauty is deceptive, however—Southwick is one of the most beastly races, thanks to the blistering heat and sandy track.

My mom and dad did their best to patch me up when we got home to Florida and insisted I take it easy—no fooling around on golf carts or daredevil stunts on the pit bikes. I maintained my fitness level with gentle cardio and kept weight training to a minimum. Injury is the one thing in life that actually slows me down—if I'm sitting down long enough to watch a television show (I like *Degrassi*), play a video game, or pick up a book, chances are it's because I'm physically incapacitated. I must have sent thousands of texts during those three weeks—my thumbs, at least, seemed to be working fine.

By the time Southwick rolled around, my back was still covered in bruises and contusions, but the broken skin had scabbed over and I was able to maneuver my left side. My wrist, having been put through the wringer this season, was still extremely fragile, and X-rays confirmed the broken bone had yet to heal fully. I knew I'd have to be extra careful not to break it again.

On race day, we lined up in the Southwick sand, sun beating down on us from an azure sky. I swatted the relentless flies from my eyes. The two-minute board went up, and I put on my helmet, glad to shield my scalp from the intense sunshine. My father's pre-race advice rang in my ears.

"Ride a safe race, Ashley. Ride smart. You've got too much to lose."

I was ahead in points for the year, and there were just two races before the end of the season, but in motocross it ain't over 'til it's over. Another injury could seriously damage my championship chances. So we had a plan—today, I wasn't riding to win. I was riding to survive.

The gate dropped and I took the holeshot, remaining in the lead for much of the opening lap—until Jessica made her way around me and took the lead. I finished the race right behind her. In the second moto I took the holeshot again, and once again it wasn't long before Jessica had caught up with me. I came in second again. Jessica had won Southwick. But with 231 points, and Jessica at 203 points, I was still ahead in the championship race. Steel City, the season finale, would be where Jessica and I faced off for the last time this season. So long as I rode sensibly and maintained the form I'd shown, the championship seemed well within reach.

Live to Laugh

There was no time to drive back to Florida in between Southwick and Steel City. (My dad, on the other hand, flew back so he could put in some time at his job. I've always been amazed that he managed to juggle a full-time job with being my coach.) So my mom, my four-year-old brother, Grandpa Motorcycle, Cody, and I cruised southwest through Connecticut toward Pittsburgh, Pennsylvania. Sarah Whitmore and her dad were following us in their motor home, as was another girl racer, Danielle Sawicki, and we had already crossed over into the Keystone State when we decided to stop at a track for some late-evening practice. We were the only people there.

The final was only four days away and I was trying hard not to worry. It had been such an intense season of expectation, pressure, and responsibility that I just wanted to feel like a teenager again. I spotted Kicker's little ten-inch X Games–branded bicycle lying on the ground beside the track, and decided to have some fun with it. Ahead of me was a shale hill, maybe fifty feet high, lit up by floodlights. I ran up the side of the hill, laughing to myself, pushing the bike in front of me along the bumpy incline. Standing at the top of the hill, the cool night breeze making me shiver just a touch, I felt more peaceful than I had in weeks. I climbed on the bike, pointed myself down the slope, and let gravity take its course. Only later did it occur to me that it probably wasn't the smartest idea, riding a five-year-old's bike down a slippery hill the night before the biggest race of my life. But I guess I can't help goofing around; I just don't like life to be boring.

Kicker's bicycle certainly wasn't built to withstand extreme outdoor mountain biking, so as I hurtled down the hill, its front end started shaking, and eventually it flipped, flinging me down to the bottom of the hill. The shale tore up my jersey sleeves, leaving some bright red road rash on my arms. My shoulder was covered in blood, and my poor wrist, which I had been taking such good care of since the X Games, was painful and swollen again. Luckily I hadn't rebroken it, but it was really tender, and I couldn't bend it.

Sarah, Cody, and Kicker couldn't believe what they had just seen. They thought it was the funniest thing ever. My mom, on the other hand, was *not* amused. We were just four days from (hopefully) wrapping up the championship, and I pulled a stunt like *this*? "Please don't tell dad!" I begged her. I knew he'd be disappointed in me for taking that kind of a risk before my last shot at winning the championship we had worked so hard for.

Steel City

Our little caravan pulled into Delmont, Pennsylvania, the day before the big race. The weather forecasts had predicted rain, so we were mentally preparing ourselves for a mud-fest, like the year before. My mom tried to reassure me: "You know you ride good in the rain, you'll be fine." In St. Augustine we get plenty of rain, so I was accustomed to showers and the steamy goggles they caused, but I couldn't help worrying. There was still a chance that Jessica could win back enough points to retain her title, and taller girls like her always have an advantage over me in the mud. They can use their legs to control themselves, whereas I'm so small, my feet don't actually reach the ground when I'm on my bike.

We checked into a somewhat dingy hotel in town, close to the track. It was jam-packed with fans and racers. As we walked through the lobby, a few amateurs stopped to ask for autographs. "You're going to win," said one girl, and I just smiled. I sure hoped she was right.

On Saturday morning, the day of the first moto, I pulled back the hotel room drapes and saw the most wonderful, perfectly blue skies I had ever seen. The showers hadn't come! It couldn't have been a more beautiful day. I thanked God for keeping the rains at bay.

At Steel City, the dirt is pretty hard packed and a little rocky. The track has a series of jumps, a triple followed by two doubles. I always hold my breath when I jump, and my heart beats really fast, so at the end of the race sometimes it feels like I've had three cardiac arrests in a row. It's only after a race that I can finally breathe normally again.

I was on my CRF250R Honda. The moments before the race are always the most tense for me, so tense I feel sick sometimes, but as soon as the gate dropped all my nerves disappeared. I took a nice clean holeshot, but Jessica wasn't going down without a fight. She knew she had to take the moto if she wanted any chance of scoring a sixth championship. She kept charging me, and it took all my strength and skill to keep her at bay. At one point she got ahead—but I didn't let her enjoy being in front for too long.

Even when I recaptured the lead, Jessica just wouldn't let up; throughout the race, I could feel her behind me, nuzzling up against my back wheel like a hungry shark chasing its prey. Then about a half a lap from the finish, the track took care of things for me. Jessica wobbled in the dirt, her front wheel slid sideways, and her bike wiped out, leaving me to cruise home with the moto. With my twenty-five points for the moto win, it was now impossible for Jessica to take the championship. I had won the series! It was over! The crowd erupted. I couldn't hear the cheers, but I could *feel* the excitement.

As soon as I dismounted I was besieged—by people giving me flowers, taking pictures, and hugging me. I saw Jessica and she gave me a thumbs-up. "Good job!" she said, and walked away. My mom and dad ran over—they both had tears in their eyes. We went back to the paddock area to decompress and by sheer coincidence, Jessica was parked next to us in the back. She was with her boyfriend, who is also her mechanic. He handed me Jessica's number one plate. "I think this belongs to you," he said.

The fact that I had won the WMA championship only started to sink in once I stood on the podium. A crowd of hundreds had gathered in front of me and they were clapping their hands, waving, and cheering. Little goose bumps broke out on my arms and I sensed they were shouting especially loud today. It all felt a little overwhelming. My experience of the world is very visual, and in front of me was an explosion of faces, camera flashes, and commotion more intense than I had ever experienced. A guy holding a microphone handed me a giant plaque with the number 1 on it. I took it from him and held it up high for everyone to see. His mouth was moving and I read his lips: "Ashley Fiolek, WMA champion!" I was the first deaf motocross champion in history.

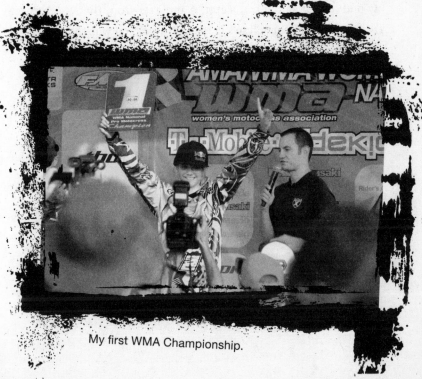

My first WMA Championship.

I had never expected to win the WMA series, not on my first try. Before that day, I had nothing to lose and nothing to prove. Now I was the national pro champion, and everything would be different. I'd have my title to lose and nothing left to prove. I was only seventeen, but in some way it felt like the end of my childhood—in less than a year I'd gone from being the deaf girl with a dream to the fastest woman on dirt.

I threw my goggles, my water bottle, and my hat into the crowd. Someone handed me a bottle of champagne and I sprayed it all over the place. I saw my parents, Kicker, Grandpa Motorcycle, and Cody out there, looking pretty much the proudest I'd ever seen them look. My dad was punching the air. We'd dreamed about this for so long.

In the white canvas media tent, I talked to the journalists, my dad acting as my translator. A reporter from the *New York Times* who had been following me that weekend was there with a cameraman. He gave me a big thumbs-up. I remember feeling proud to even be at a press conference. This felt like Christmas—better than Christmas—and all my birthdays rolled into one. A whoosh of images—broken bones, riding in Wolverine Forest, Grandpa Motorcycle smiling—all exploded in my mind. It felt like my journey, starting with riding my PW50 bike through the woods in Michigan, was flashing in front of me. This is what everything had been pointing toward. *Today.*

That night we went back to the hotel, too exhausted to celebrate anymore. I slept harder than I had in months.

The next day I still had to race the second moto—but it was a mere formality at this point as I already had all the points I needed to win the championship. I could concentrate on actually having some fun. The gate dropped and I took the holeshot.

Not long after Jessica pulled around me, and then Tarah. The two of them duked it out in front of me. Tarah ended up winning her first moto of the season, and I was happy for her. I came in third in that moto. But I was twenty-nine points ahead of Jessica Patterson overall, and won the championship.

That night, I was in the mood to celebrate. A group of WMA girls, Miki, and my family and I headed to a Pittsburgh restaurant called Smokey Bones. After such a tense season, everyone was ready to let off some steam—and I don't think the restaurant knew what they were in for. Toward the end of the meal, as a joke, I took some whipped cream from my pie and dabbed it on the nose of one of the moms sitting next to me. Tarah Gieger pointed at Cody with a wicked glint in her eye. I flung a handful of whipped cream at Cody, narrowly missing him but hitting my agent—*thunk*—in the middle of his forehead. After that, our table descended into chaos, with everyone flinging food and Kicker racing around the table like a lunatic. The Smokey Bones manager threatened to kick us out, but nobody seemed to be paying much attention. It's a moment I'll never forget. And I don't think they will either.

R&R

Back in St. Augustine, I gave myself a couple months to relax—time off is *really* important to me. The way I see it, taking time out just helps make me more hungry to win. After not being on a dirt bike for a while, I start craving it. Time out also gives me a chance to reflect. What did this all mean? Now that I was the WMA champion, where was I supposed to go from here? When I wanted to switch off my thoughts, I would make little movies—

sometimes poor Kicker would get to star in them, and I'd dress him up in funny costumes, making him look like a rapper, with jewelry and a backward baseball cap. Universal Studios and Disney World are just a few hours' drive away, so I went there and checked out the roller coasters. Sarah had gotten me into roller coasters—when we went to MGM Studios one time, she joked that if I didn't go on the roller coaster with her, she'd write that I was a big wimp in her magazine column. So of course, I got on, and now I can't get enough of crazy fairground rides.

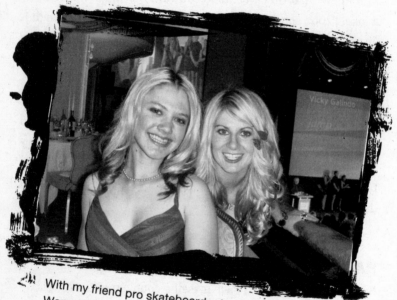

With my friend pro skateboarder Lyn-Z Hawkins, at the 2008 Women's Sports Foundation's benefit dinner at the Waldorf Astoria Hotel in New York.

After winning the WMA, I made the cover of *TransWorld Motocross* magazine, the first woman racer to do so. The two

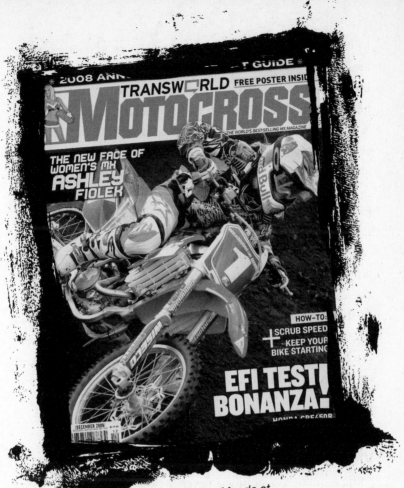

Courtesy of Donn Maeda at TransWorld Motocross magazine.

biggest motocross magazines are *TransWorld* and *Racer X,* and Donn Maeda, the editor of *TransWorld,* had been a supporter of mine for a long while. He even invited me to write a monthly column for them, "Silence."

And the coverage wasn't limited to motocross publications—all kinds of magazines and newspapers wanted to talk to me now. *Rolling Stone,* the *New York Times,* and *Paper* magazine. That's how I met Caroline, the journalist who wrote this book with me—through *Paper* magazine. She thought what was happening in women's motocross was interesting and believed it was a story more people needed to hear. It was heartening, seeing people who might never have given motocross a second glance starting to take an interest in this world.

Many publications seemed to be especially intrigued by the fact that I am deaf. I had to become skilled at giving interviews with my parents translating. There aren't many journalists who can sign, and we do a lot of interviews on the phone. Sometimes it feels like I do more interviewing than training. But it's part of the job, and I'm always happy to tell the world about what I do. To this day, I believe my deafness, while on the surface defined as a handicap, has helped me in ways I could never have imagined. I've had to be tougher and work harder than hearing folks. And my deafness has made people pay more attention to the sport than they would have if I was a regular, hearing girl.

Victim of Motocross

Being a motocross family is never easy. For so long, 99 percent of our lives had been focused on me—me racing a dirt bike and me getting better at it. There were so many money issues and sponsorship issues and motocross issues that other things—like the health of my parents' marriage—had been pushed to the sidelines.

My mom and dad—Roni and Jim from Dearborn, Michigan—had always believed that God had given them a girl with a talent, a deaf girl with a talent, and that it was their duty to help that talent grow to its maximum potential. But the constant traveling, the lack of privacy, the worrying about money—after a while it all became too much to bear. I think they just both got tired.

When my parents told me and Kicker that they were splitting up, I was sad, but the announcement didn't come as a huge surprise. They had been living relatively separate lives for a while—my mom staying home with Kicker, my dad training with me on the road. I tried to be as understanding as I could, although I worried that maybe it was my fault.

"It's got *nothing* to do with you or Kicker," my mom reassured me. "These are issues between me and your dad." They explained that sometimes love isn't enough for people to make a marriage work. It takes time and effort and communication, and they'd allowed themselves to neglect one another as they helped me fulfill my motocross dream. They promised me that things were going to carry on as they always had, in terms of my motocross. I wanted them both to be happy and all of us to keep working together, but I accepted that some things would have to change.

My dad decided he would move into the motor home and park it in an RV park close to our home while he and my mom figured out the next steps. Kicker was pretty upset—he didn't want my dad to leave. But ours was an all-too-common story—each year young athletes' families break up because of the pressures. Some motocross parents have had to remortgage their home two or three times just to support their kids' racing. You can imagine the toll that takes on everyone. Suddenly we had to face the possibility that the Fioleks, too, would become a motocross statistic.

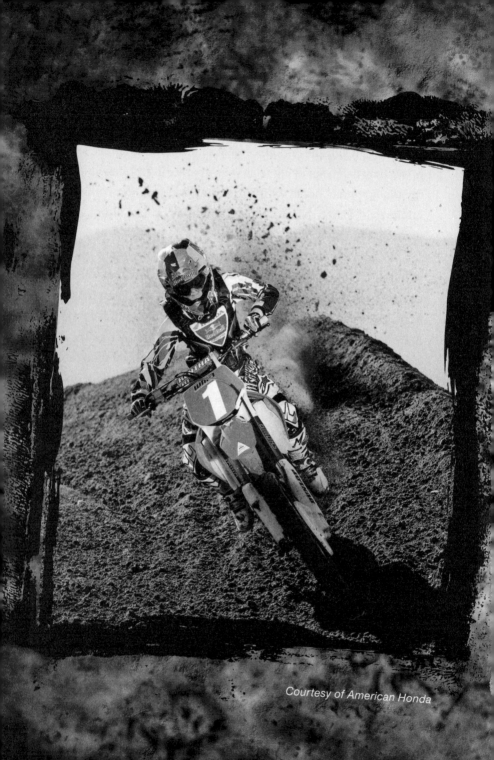

Courtesy of American Honda

Cody seemed less enthusiastic—unlike me, he's not always hungry. "You guys go, and I'll stay here and look after Kicker," he said.

But my mom wasn't taking no for an answer. "No, you should be there, Cody. We need to talk about next year's plans." Both Cody and I stiffened—what did she mean? My dad wanted us to meet him at an Outback Steakhouse nearby. Cody fidgeted the whole way there—I could tell he was nervous. I was in the passenger seat next to my mom, and she seemed very focused on the road. *Something's going on,* I thought.

We walked into the steakhouse and found my dad. He had already ordered some drinks and appetizers. We sat down, and after a few minutes' small talk my mom started rummaging around her handbag, pulling out a piece of paper with something printed on it. She handed it to me.

"This is what your next motorcycle is going to look like," she said. I looked at the cut-out—it was a top-of-the-line Honda works bike, the kind the factory boys ride. I didn't get it. I looked at Cody, and he seemed just as confused. My mom and dad started laughing. "Ashley, this is *your* bike," said my dad. "It's brand-new." A brand-new factory bike, for me? This could only mean one thing—*was I really on the Honda Factory team?* I was stunned and thrilled. No woman in American motocross had ever been invited to join a factory team before.

I had so many questions, it was hard to know where to begin. How had this come about, how long had they known, were they *sure*? I had no idea that Honda was considering making me the fifth member of their elite factory team. It turned out my agent and parents had been talking with reps from the major bike companies all year long. After my WMA performance and the

chapter 8

FACTORY GIRL

Trip to the Outback

November in St. Augustine—I loved this time of year. The oppressive humidity of the summer months had eased and finally I could breathe without having to blast the AC all the time. The motocross season was over, and it was time to regroup, relax, and make plans for the following year. Ordinarily, my dad would light fires out in the back and invite his buddies over when the nights started getting cool. Now he was living in the motor home, and the house felt quieter. He came over to visit plenty, but still—I missed him.

One afternoon Cody and I were hanging out, playing with Kicker, when my mom called us over. "Your dad and I want to take you for dinner," she signed.

"Sure," I said. When it comes to eating out, you don't have t twist my arm. "Where are we going?" There was something ten in her manner. I could tell she was holding something back, b I didn't know what.

attention that brought, Honda had decided to make me an offer. My parents had been negotiating for months but hadn't said a word about it. "We didn't want to distract you from your racing," said my dad. "And honestly, we didn't want you to feel let down if it didn't work out."

The waitress came by to take our orders and I asked for the biggest steak on the menu—this called for a celebration! The first person we called was Donn Maeda from *TransWorld*. "Oh, I had a feeling this was in the cards," he said. "I've been telling Honda for years you needed to be on their factory team."

My mom was holding the phone, talking to him, acting as a conversational go-between. "Well, looks like they might have listened to you, Donn," I signed.

Being on a factory team meant that finally my family would be relieved of the financial burden of paying for me to get to races. From now on, Honda Red Bull Racing would cover hotel rooms and flights for me and Cody. My dad would actually be able to keep the money he made from his job, rather than spending it all on me. We formed a company from which I would draw a salary and pay for my family's travel expenses. Honda would give me parts and fix my bike. Finally, I was going to make a living—a good one—out of racing a motorcycle. That day's news was a sign that the tide was really starting to turn for female racers.

Golden State

In December 2008, Honda invited me to their facility in Torrance, California. There, I would be officially introduced to my new factory teammates Andrew Short, Ivan Tedesco, Ben Townley, and Davi Millsaps. I had grown up racing with Davi in Florida, and when he saw me, he stopped in his tracks. "No way! It's *you*," said Davi, beaming. Honda Red Bull had told the boys that there was going to be a new addition to the team but they hadn't said it was going to be a girl.

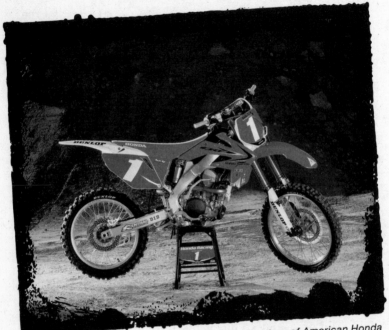

My new ride. *Courtesy of American Honda*

Testing, Testing

We set to work testing my bike right away, seeing how it responded to my body, build, and riding style under every imaginable set of conditions. If I didn't like the way my bike was reacting to anything I would tell the team of Honda mechanics and they would adjust it and cut it down. The aim was to make the bike and me run like one entity. Cody was still on board, washing my bike, changing tires, and greasing things up, but now I had a whole new team of super mechanics too, one looking after my engine, another in charge of my suspension, another for my chassis—as many as ten dedicated technicians for just five factory racers. We'd test the bike at various tracks, under different conditions—one time, Honda rented the entire Glen Helen track so its factory riders could test!

Because of all the testing, Honda encouraged us to move to California for the next five or so months, so I could be based close to their workshop. There, they could get my bike into tip-top condition while I prepared for the next WMA season, the X Games, and the European grand prix races. It seemed to make sense—my mom, Kicker, and I would find a house in California, and my dad would stay back in Florida, and carry on working his job.

Honda decided to tell the rest of the world about their newest factory rider—me—at the official opening of the Red Bull training facility, a month or so later. It made sense, as all the motorsports press and industry top brass would be there.

By the time I arrived, the place was buzzing with media. And when the Honda officials called them in for a press conference, I could tell many of the journalists were more than a little surprised to see a tiny blond girl wearing the factory Honda jersey. By the end of the day, though, they seemed almost as excited as we were. This marked the start of a new era in women's motocross!

I was presented with my new ride: Honda's CRF250R, even though I was riding on a 450 team. (Girls aren't actually permitted to ride 450 dirt bikes at pro races—a 250 is as high as we could go. For my height and weight, I'm more than happy on a 250.) Immediately after the party, the team started customizing

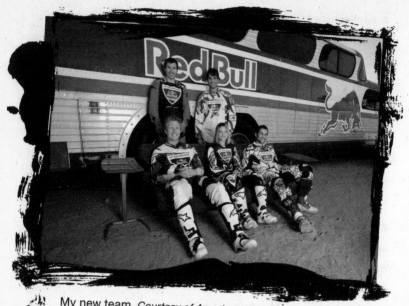

My new team. *Courtesy of American Honda*

it, shortening the frame, cutting the seat down, and trimming the handlebars for me because I'm so tiny. As a factory rider, I now had a team of experts available to me, experts whose sole job it was to ensure that my bike was *exactly* as I needed it. At races, they would be at my disposal, working on everything from my motor to my chassis to my suspension. There was a whole village behind me now, it seemed.

The bikes themselves were unlike anything I had ridden before. I was always the type of kid who would ride anything—even if the handlebars were mangled, I'd hop on. Now I was riding bikes whose suspension alone could cost $75,000. Riding prototype machines added a whole new dimension to my life in motocross. Along with practicing and racing, testing would now be a big part of my life.

A Big Girl Now

My dad has always wanted nothing but the best for me. He's demanded perfection, as have I. To be a good motocross coach you *have* to be tough. But having Jim Fiolek be my coach *and* my father had become confusing. I wanted my father back.

We had talked about it regularly over the years—in fact, my dad had offered to stop coaching me several times but I hadn't felt ready to separate from him. The tension between us was part of the reason we had brought in trainers to work with me, like Ronnie Tichenor and Shannon Niday. We hoped they would take the pressure off and give us the space we needed to build a normal father-daughter relationship. But I always ended up asking him to be my coach again. No one else could communicate with me the way he did. No trainers knew sign language. Quite simply, I needed my father there. He knew me and what I was capable of, what I could and couldn't do. We had a language that no one else understood.

In the end, there was no earth-shattering moment, no monumental argument that led to our parting ways as athlete and coach—like my parents' separation, this was something that had been building up for years. But now, in February of 2009, taking some space just seemed to make sense. We both felt it was for the best. It was a strange time for me. My parents' relationship was on the rocks, my dependence on my father was dissolving. I was in emotional free fall.

I soon found out it wasn't easy flying solo. You have to push yourself. You have to be organized and plan your own strategy. I was used to my dad telling me when to practice, when to ride, where to ride, how much to ride—I had to start doing all that on my own.

Leaving my father behind in Florida while the rest of us moved to California wasn't easy. "I wish I could be the person who helps you go faster," my dad told me as we said good-bye. My mom and Kicker were waiting in the truck, and there were tears in his eyes.

"You are, Dad," I signed. "You always have been."

California Dreamin'

After our California visit in January, we had about three months to prepare ourselves for the big move. We returned the Monday after Easter, headed for our new home in Riverside County—the spiritual home of motocross. We wanted to spend around half of the year there, and our good friend Rick Wernli, a devoted member of the motocross clan who had been my mechanic on and off, offered to help us get settled. He found us a house in Canyon Lake, a pretty, gated lakeside community with fourteen miles of shoreline. Best of all, it was within a forty-five-minute drive of some of the region's best tracks—Perris Raceway, Glen Helen, Competitive Edge Raceway, Starwest, and Pala Raceway.

Even though the last two or three years have seen more of the motocross industry relocate to Florida or Texas, SoCal is generally where it's at in my sport. The epicenter is southwest Riverside County between Corona and Temecula, about an hour and a half east of L.A. Top men pros like Ricky Johnson and Broc Glover came from there, specifically from the El Cajon area (they call it the "El Cajon Zone"). Go to any popular open riding area on any given day in our new home base, and you'd most likely find ten to fifteen major pro racers out there training. Supercross heroes Jeremy McGrath, Chad Reed, and James Stewart had homes in the area, as did my friend E-Bash—now we were neighbors.

Motocross flourished in this part of the world partially because it's where all the factories are based. Honda is in Torrance, Yamaha is in Buena Park, Suzuki is in Fullerton, and Kawasaki is in Irvine. And when the factories need to test bikes, they can take them into the wide open spaces of Riverside County.

As soon as we unpacked, I felt at home. We had a defined plan—my mom, Kicker, and Cody would stay in Canyon Lake from April until August, when the X Games ended. We would fly to all the races, except those in California, which we would drive to. My dad would fly in from Florida to meet us. There was something about the openness, the golden hills, and the dry heat that made me feel optimistic. California felt like the perfect place for us to be at that moment, and the more time I spent there (did I mention how great the sushi restaurants are in California?), the more seriously I started considering moving there permanently. My main reason for being in Florida had been to go to school—and I hadn't been in school for years. California was winning me over.

Don't Leave Your Golf Carts Unattended

The spring and summer of 2009 E-Bash and I got to hang out more than we ever had. Three or four times a week, we would drive to a track or hang at each others' houses playing with our dogs. She has two chocolate Labs, Buster and Missy, and Kicker and I have two English bulldogs, Turbo and Rocco. We usually practiced together at Perris Raceway, Competitive Edge, and Glen Helen. Riding with her is always fun, because we have such different riding styles—she's smooth and more cautious than I am. If someone is passing her she'll let that person go, whereas I'm more aggressive. Like the time we raced Steel City together and I bumped E-bash getting out of the gate.

"Why did you do that?" she asked me afterward. It would never be her style to bump into anyone.

"Why? Because it's a race!" I signed back, nonplussed.

Golf carts and rental cars—two things you should never leave unattended when there are motocross racers around. You can pretty much guarantee they will come back wrecked. One of our favorite pastimes was to drive golf carts around and try to jump them. Aside from just goofing around it was comforting to me having a good friend like her around. I knew I had a lot to prove this season, and I was going to need all the support I could get.

Gearing Up for the New Season

Some important changes were in place for 2009. There were opportunities for women professional racers that just hadn't been there before—this year we would get an eight-stop series alongside the men at the nationals, and equal money at the X Games. Finally we would be able to park in the same area as the guys. We were going to get timed qualifiers and more TV time. (Outdoor motocross is very hard to get on live television because of the amount of work and structure that goes into laying the mile and a half of cable necessary to broadcast a race.)

I was pleased with the two extra races on the schedule— two more races than last year, at Glen Helen Raceway in San Bernardino and High Point Raceway in Mount Morris, Pennsylvania. Then there were the other tracks we had raced last year—Hangtown, Freestone, Thunder Valley, Washougal, South-wick, and Steel City. Going into the 2009 season I was ranked number one, Jessica was number two, and Sarah was number three. Tarah was number four and my buddy E-Bash was ranked number seven. I had heard that Jessica had stepped up her training and lost weight. The way I see it, competition is always a good thing—it pushes us to be our very best. So when I heard how hard Jessica was working, it was the perfect motivator. Some of the motocross media were even starting to say there was an "epic championship battle" ahead.

The 2009 season was going to be a nail-biter.

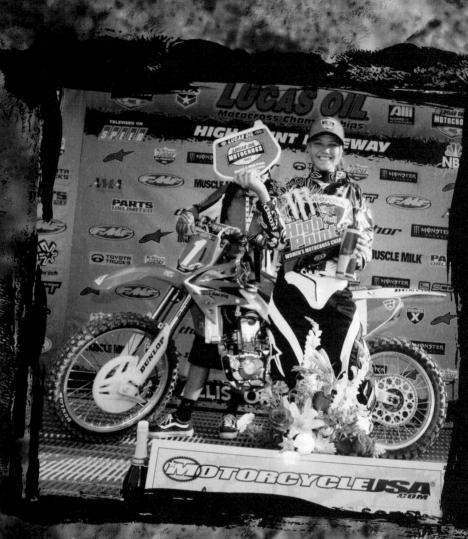
On the podium at High Point. *Carl Stone*

chapter 9

SUMMER OF RECKONING

Glen Helen

It was another dry, perfectly cloudless morning in Southern California, and May was drawing to a close. My dad had flown in from Florida a couple days earlier, and Grandpa Motorcycle had driven across the country so he could join us for the first race of the season. At around six A.M. we packed up our truck and set off from the house in Canyon Lake, all together, heading north up the 15 freeway toward the San Bernardino National Forest. An hour later we arrived at the infamous Glen Helen Raceway, occasional site of heavy metal festivals like Ozzfest (in 2005 the heavy metal band Iron Maiden was famously pelted with eggs by fans at Glen Helen), where today, the 2009 motocross season was officially kicking off.

We pulled into the parched, sprawling site, dust clouds billowing behind the trailer truck. We trundled toward the pit area and parked. The land was arid and almost entirely devoid of vegetation. We saw Travis Pastrana with his girlfriend, my fellow pro racer Sherri Cruse. And there was the Honda Red Bull Racing rig, with its cordoned-off warm-up area and shiny semi-trailer truck. Inside, each of the factory racers had their own bunk. There we could get dressed, pray, or simply relax in solitude. It felt incredibly deluxe compared to the motor home—like a hotel suite on the dirt.

Cody was already there, working on my bike. Now that I was a factory racer, my bike traveled everywhere on the Honda rig. Miki was there too, as were most of the other pro racers, male and female, working on their bikes and setting up. Fans were already trickling in, and a line of SUVs, trucks, and RVs snaked back from the entrance gateway—twenty thousand or so people had bought tickets at $40 a pop to watch us race today.

Both fans and racers were adjusting to some sweeping changes—the biggest being that Davey Coombs's MX Sports had taken over promoting the pro championship from the AMA. Miki had sold the WMA National Championship to MX Sports, and the WMA would now be known as the WMX. We hoped this partnership meant that things were going to be different.

This year men and women would be racing on the same day (before, women raced once on Saturday and once on Sunday). This was the first time the WMX races were to be included as part of the main program, meaning thousands more fans would be watching women's racing this year. There was no denying that men's racing was still, at the end of the day, the biggest draw. But this year, at least the fans would have the opportunity to check out what we women were doing. And hopefully they'd like what they saw.

The track itself, a circuit of steep, rutted hills and treacherous hairpins, had been entirely refurbished, and hundreds of tons of sand were brought in to create a brand-new whoops section. The lineup included a handful of promising new women rookies who, like me the year before, had just graduated from the amateur ranks into pro racing.

Now that I was a factory racer, I was constantly on display, both on and off the track. Some fans pay extra to have access to the pit area so they can watch their favorite riders get ready. I tried not to feel self-conscious as I warmed up my muscles on the stationary bikes in front of the rig, pedaling in front of dozens of onlookers. "This is part of your job now," my dad reminded me. "People have paid all this money to be here, so they want to get as close to the athletes as they can."

The first women's moto at Glen Helen was also the first race of the day, at around one P.M. I put on my neck brace and chest protector as the Honda mechanics, five of them, rapidly updated me on the state of the bike and how best to ride it under the day's conditions. My dad was translating and I nodded as I took it all in. I was glad to have him there.

I kissed my helmet, put it on, and climbed on my dirt bike, which was gleaming. Cody climbed on the back with me and we rode through the pits, crowds parting as we headed toward the starting line. Fans saw my number one plate and gave us the thumbs-up, smiling as we passed. We drove past sponsor kiosks with show bikes suspended in the air, girls in bikinis posing for photos, the smell of hot dogs and popcorn. People from all over the state, the country, the *world* had gathered to see us race. There was so much color, vibration, and movement—what I see at races certainly *feels* "loud" and intense. We neared the track—people were climbing all over the sidelines like ants, picking their spot in the dust, camping out with the family on chairs and under umbrellas to protect themselves from the relentless midday sun. I knew my mom and Kicker were out there, somewhere, waiting for the race to begin.

Waiting at the line, my CRF250R bike felt huge, but I felt more than confident that I could control it. On top of an intense few months of training, I had been on a specialized nutrition and exercise regime with my trainer Robb, and my strength was way up. Jessica, my main competition for this season, had been training with an ex–motocross racer who had a reputation for pushing his protégées to the limit. Word was that her form was better than ever.

I lined up among the twenty-five or so girl pros next to me. Cody held an umbrella over my head to shield me from the sun. Kids clung to wire fencing watching us—little boys with dirty faces and their motocross hats on backward—and I remembered once feeling like they did, like a fan in awe of the racers. Cody gave me a hug and left, and it was just us girls, looking straight ahead and waiting for the gate to drop.

I saw the two-minute board and cleared my mind, waiting for the gate to drop. I rocketed out of the starting gate to claim the holeshot by a very comfortable lead—a great way to start the 2009 season. The circuit was rough, tough, and hard packed, and speeding around the first corner I reminded myself to keep calm and not make any dumb mistakes. Overconfidence, underconfidence—both are the enemy of a motocross racer.

The sun was high up in the sky and shadows were visible but short. It was hard to tell who, if anyone, was coming up behind me but nobody ever did. I nailed the moto and punched the air as I flew across the finish line, the checkered flag waving behind me. The second moto of the day went almost exactly the same way—holeshot, followed by a lead, although Jessica was close behind me at the finish. A solid victory on one of the toughest tracks in America!

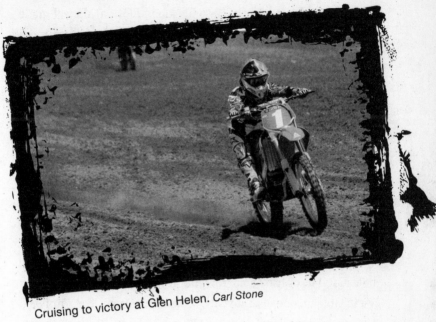
Cruising to victory at Glen Helen. *Carl Stone*

I was glad to have gotten Glen Helen out of the way. I knew there were people watching who wondered if last season's win was a fluke. Maybe this would put their doubts to rest.

Hanging on at Hangtown

The Friday after Glen Helen, my mom, my dad, Kicker, and I drove in our truck out of Canyon Lake again, winding our way north, up the Golden State Freeway into Northern California. Hangtown, the track near Sacramento, was our destination.

My dad had flown in from Florida so we could drive up to-gether and spend some time as a family; at times like these, it felt like nothing much had changed. It was easy to pretend that my parents weren't really separating—until the end of the weekend, when my dad would fly back to his job in Florida, alone. I made the most of having him around and noticed that he and my mom seemed more relaxed around each other than they had been in a long while. The separation, and having my dad step down as my coach, seemed to have eased the pressure-cooker atmosphere that had followed us around the last twelve years.

The track at Hangtown was looking great to me—neither dusty nor muddy. Normally the weather is a little cooler up there than it is in SoCal—but not on race day. Once again I thanked the Lord for making me immune to the extremes of heat and cold, because everyone around me was complaining about global warming and how uncomfortable they were.

I set the pace once again in the first moto and claimed the holeshot, but only by a narrow margin. Right up behind me was Vicki Golden, one of that year's rookie sensations. But I finished the moto unchallenged with a 4.39-second lead. The main battle was going on behind me, between Vicki and Jessica Patterson.

For a while, it seemed like the second moto would play out in much the same way as the first—the holeshot was mine, and this time I had Jessica right behind me instead of Vicki. Then Jes-sica made her way in front of me—and she wasn't giving me any opportunity to reclaim my lead. We battled all the way to the finish, my bike not handling the jumps as well as I had hoped. I knew this time I wouldn't be able to catch up. I won Hangtown overall on points, but my mechanics weren't happy.

"Your suspension needs some work," said my technician, grim faced. In the short week between Hangtown and the next race—at Freestone in Texas—they took my bike back to the Honda shop and tore it apart, completely reworking the suspension. After repeated testing on my part, it was race-ready and back on the road—destination, Texas. I waved good-bye to my bike as it set off on the next leg of its journey on the Honda rig.

Freestone—No Margin for Error

Freestone County Raceway lies in the tiny town of Wortham, Texas (population one thousand), an hour and a half south of Dallas and the highest point between Dallas and Houston. Freestone was among the newer tracks in the series, founded ten years prior and with just three years of pro racing to its name. The environment couldn't have been more different from Hangtown's—Wortham is flat as a pancake compared with the steep rolling hills that surround Hangtown. My mom, Cody, Kicker, and I flew to Dallas and checked into a hotel that Honda had booked for us. I thought back to the days in the motor home, rushing to get to the next race with the bike behind us, and smiled. We'd certainly come a long way.

This would be the second time we women had raced at Freestone, and it wasn't going to be an easy ride. The track made up for its flatness with some intense turns. This was going to require a very clear head. There was no margin for error. *Keep it together, Ashley,* I thought as we lined up at the starting gate. I took my fifth holeshot in a row and before long, Jessica and I had pushed ahead and resumed our ongoing battle, with the other riders at a safe distance behind us. Jessica was trying to get past me at each treacherous turn, but I kept her at bay. I knew so long as I kept my cool, things would be fine. I saw the white flag, indicating we were on the final lap—victory was within my grasp. I relaxed a little—and of course as soon as I did, Jessica seized her chance: I felt a *whoosh* as she squeezed ahead of me, taking me by surprise.

A set of sand whoops lay ahead of us—the only way I could possibly reclaim my lead would be to throw caution to the wind and take a different line into them, a line no one else had used. I pulled on the throttle and hurtled into the whoops, clinging on for dear life. Before long, Jessica was behind me again. I'd stolen back the moto!

Afterward I headed back to the trailer and splashed my face with water. I thanked God for being on my side, and keeping me safe. Did I really win again? I guess so.

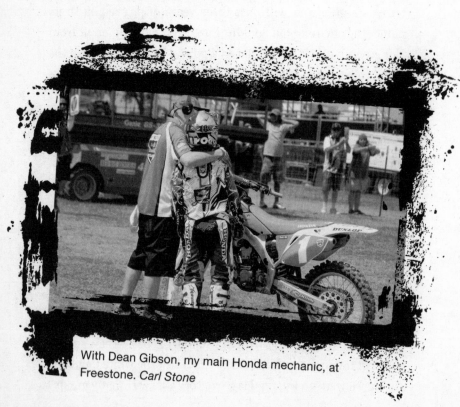

With Dean Gibson, my main Honda mechanic, at Freestone. *Carl Stone*

In the next moto Jessica suffered some bad luck—after crashing in the first turn she lost valuable minutes trying to restart her bike and never really made it back into the race. Meanwhile, I found myself with another battle on my hands—Sara Price, a rookie rider, was head-to-head with me for the first few laps until she lost momentum and I pushed ahead. I was looking forward to racing her again—she had given me a run for my money! But the second moto and the race were mine.

High Hopes at High Point

The next race, at High Point Raceway in Mount Morris, Pennsylvania, marked the midway point of the season. The track, close to the West Virginia state line, has been raced since 1976. But this year its owner, the formidable Davey Coombs, had hired one of the top track builders in the world to create some new jump combinations designed to thrill both the riders and the fans.

The track has an uphill start and Sherri Cruse, one of the top five WMX pros, broke my run of holeshot wins, speeding away ahead of everyone else as the gate dropped. Jessica and I were right behind her. Then Jessica pushed past Sherri aggressively, forcing her off the track and stealing the lead. I soon drew up close behind her and by the time we went around the second lap, I was in the lead. Behind me, Jessica suffered more bad luck and dropped way back after she lost control and fell. She was only able to make it back to fourth position.

We returned to the track that evening for the second moto, with the sun low in the sky. It was cooler, in the mid-seventies, but the atmosphere was just as heated as it had been earlier in the day. This time around I took the holeshot and, after another battle with Jessica, won the race comfortably. I already had a thirty-four-point lead over Jessica in the series. Could I possibly dream of winning the WMX Championship twice in a row?

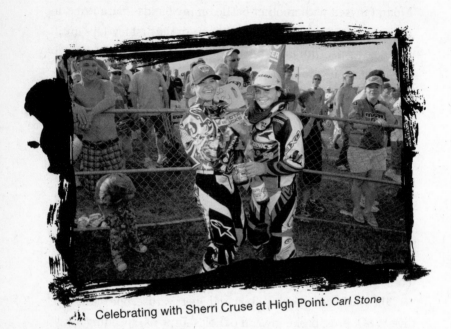
Celebrating with Sherri Cruse at High Point. *Carl Stone*

Storming Thunder Valley

We went back to Thunder Valley, Colorado, in the foothills of the Rocky Mountains, just west of Denver. With the 6,100-foot elevation, racing there feels like racing in the clouds. My Honda mechanics were busily adjusting the jetting on my bike so it would run well in this heavenly race environment.

We arrived a few days early to thunder storms in Thunder Valley, typical for late June. Thankfully by the time race day rolled around, the skies had cleared and conditions were pretty much perfect. I was starting to wonder if we had guardian angels in the clouds, taking care of the weather for us.

Thunder Valley is the only track where racing takes place at night, with giant floodlights that illuminate the soft mountainside dirt. Night riding is always a little surreal—particularly with fireworks and flamethrowers going off all around the track. I won the two motos at Thunder Valley but both were hard fought, this time with the Brazilian racer Mariana Balbi banging my handlebars all the way to the checkers in moto two. As fireworks shot up into the night sky and tumbled like shooting stars, marking the end of the race, I reveled in the knowledge that I was on a winning streak—what could go wrong?

Taking on Horsepower Hill

At the foot of the Cascade Mountains in the Pacific Northwest, about an hour from Portland, Oregon, is Washougal. Green, woodsy, and magical, with pine trees and fir trees all around, this is where the *Twilight* movies were filmed. And the track there is among my favorites in the country, with massive changes in elevation, fast riding conditions, and spectacular vistas. The Japanese national women's champion Haruna Masu had flown out to Washougal especially to race against us, and I was ready to tear up the hillsides with a fresh challenger on the track.

The Pacific Northwest is usually cool and temperate—we just happened to arrive in the middle of one of the biggest heat waves to ever hit the region. It was nearly 100 degrees in the shade on race day, with hardly any breeze. Again, I didn't let the heat affect me and tapped into my inner ice box, remembering the freezing-cold Michigan winters. In the first moto, I sped out the gate and took the holeshot. Ahead of me was Horsepower Hill, one of the toughest obstacles in American motocross, a huge uphill. But riders can't allow fearful thoughts to creep in during a race; that's suicide! I cleared the hill, my mind only on keeping Jessica from taking the lead. Luckily my hard work paid off—the moto was mine.

In the second moto, Haruna, the Japanese racer, took the holeshot, while Jessica amped up the aggression, nudging me and trying to knock me down. I found myself in fourth place and had to battle to get into third, and then second place behind Jessica, but her lead was too strong. Jessica took the second moto and won Washougal—my first real defeat of the season.

Standing on the podium in second place, I didn't allow myself to feel too disappointed—I knew I still had a comfortable points lead in the championship. So long as I kept my cool, the trophy was well within reach.

Walking the Red Rug

In June I found out I had been nominated for an ESPN ESPY award—kind of like the Grammys or Oscars of the sports world. I had been nominated in the Best Female Action Sports Athlete category, which American snowboarder Gretchen Bleiler had won the year before. The awards ceremony was held in the middle of July at the Nokia Theatre in downtown Los Angeles, with Samuel L. Jackson hosting. Other nominees included NBA star LeBron James and tennis champion Serena Williams—an A-list lineup. Racing on mud, covered in dirt and sweaty, I never once imagined that a red carpet would find its way into my life.

The night before, my mom, Kicker, Cody, and I checked into the Standard Hotel, where we had booked a room. "Is this for swingers?" my mom joked as we peered inside our ultra-modern room. The bed had no frame and the bathroom—and shower—

had no doors, just glass walls. The four of us looked at one another giggling. We weren't nudists, so this was going to take some delicate maneuvering.

The hotel was also hosting the ESPY gifting suites, where companies that wanted to give us free products would set up shop. It felt like Christmas . . . I loaded up with gifts in room upon room, smiling people handing us bags containing all kinds of stuff we never knew we needed—like a new showerhead, for example. And deodorants, duffle bags, clothes, necklaces, candles, incense, DVDs, coffee, pillowcases, and bottles of wine that I was too young to drink. In one room I got my hair and makeup done for the red carpet by Bobbi Brown stylists. They gave me the biggest 'do I had ever had, and I didn't mind it at all—when you spend most of your life covered in dirt, it feels good to be pampered once in a while.

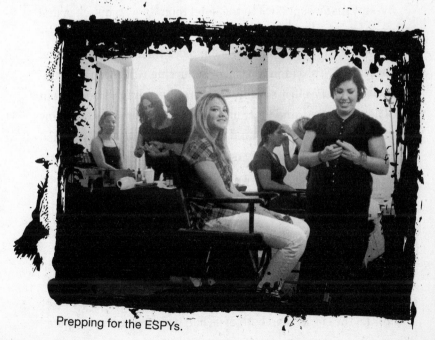

Prepping for the ESPYs.

My mom was my date for the ceremony (Cody stayed at the hotel and watched Kicker). I was wearing a purple dress and high heels—I couldn't remember the last time I had worn heels—and smiling as hard as I could for the cameras. Every famous athlete you could think of was there—I spotted Michael Phelps and Shawn Johnson—talking to reporters on the red carpet before making their way inside the Nokia Theatre auditorium. What a night!

I had been nominated for the Best Female Action Sports Athlete award, alongside three other girls: snowboarder Torah Bright, skier Sarah Burke, and Maya Gabeira, a Brazilian big-wave surfer, who ended up winning. Only a handful of motocrossers have been nominated for an ESPY before—Travis Pastrana, Ricky Carmichael, Jessica Patterson, and James Stewart—so it was a huge honor.

The after-party was at a Lucky Strike bowling alley close by—my mom went back to the hotel room to watch Kicker, and Cody came out to join me for the festivities. The after party was packed with people, most of them older than us, drinking and partying. We stood in a corner, wondering what we were supposed to do. We felt so silly, we started giggling. "Let's get out of here," I signed, and Cody nodded. Back at our shiny hotel, my mom and Kicker were sound asleep in the room. Cody passed out immediately. I got into my pajamas, threw my purple dress on top of the bags of gifts in the corner, and lay back on the bed, thinking of mud.

X Marks the Spot

It was July and E-Bash and I were at the house in Canyon Lake, sitting in the backyard as the sun set. The X Games were right around the corner, and both of us had been invited to compete.

"I really hope I get to go," I signed. E-Bash nodded. Now that I was a factory rider, there was a chance Honda might not even allow me to compete. The X Games is such an injury-fest, factories are often nervous about exposing their top riders to the risk—especially right in the middle of the championship series. My teammates Davi Millsaps and Ivan Tedesco had already been told they wouldn't be allowed to enter by top Honda brass in Japan. "They probably won't let you compete either," one of my mechanics at the Red Bull facility told me. "They don't want you to damage yourself and throw away the championship."

But my agent told me to stop worrying. "Ashley, we had it written in your contract specifically that you should be allowed to enter the X Games. You'll be there."

I felt like Cinderella opening her invitation to the ball.

Upon hearing the news, my mechanics at Honda set to work on my suspension, making sure it could withstand the unforgiving X Games supercross track that awaited me. I was so ready!

Soon enough it was the last weekend in July, the weekend of the X Games, and I was more than ready to make up for my no-show the year before. This year the stakes were high—the prize money for women had been quadrupled to $40,000, the same as the boys.

Once again, the track had been built in the Home Depot Center in Carson, an open-air sports complex that's home to the Los Angeles Galaxy soccer team. As usual, it featured steep triple jumps, a big finish-line jump, and earth so hard it had become what we call "blue grooved"—when earth is so compacted it turns blue from the black of the tires. My family and I had already decided ahead of time that I wasn't going to take any unnecessary risks at the X Games. I didn't want to destroy myself either. We talked it over as a family and decided I should race smart, race cautious. I practiced a few days ahead of the race on Saturday, getting a chance to fully experience the track's viciousness. I crashed badly on the huge finish-line jump, smacking my head so hard on the earth I was seeing stars and landing on my hand so badly I thought I had broken all my fingers. It was a sobering practice session.

The X Games take place over three days, which allowed us plenty of time to ooh and aah at the amazing extreme athletes who were competing. My mom, Miki, and I went down to the bleachers to watch my friend Lyn-Z Hawkins, a pro skateboarder, compete. We sat down just in time to see Lyn-Z's final competition. There was no shade whatsoever on what felt like the hottest L.A. day ever. Our clothes were drenched in sweat as we watched Lyn-Z do her run of skate tricks. "Wow—she's really shredding!" I signed, marveling. The judges added up the scores and sure enough, Lyn-Z had won gold at the X Games, for the third time in her career.

She was awarded her medal on a podium set up in the middle of the ramp. Afterward she saw us and came running over, smiling wide. She pressed her medal into my hand. "Feel it, girl," she said. My mom and I looked at one another. Seeing the look on Lyn-Z's face and feeling the medal in my palm—well, I had to go for it now. I started signing. "OK, Mom—I'm going to go for gold!" So much for playing it safe.

Going for Gold

That was Thursday—on Saturday, it was my turn in the stadium. Our race was due to take place late, at six fifteen or so, after the boys had finished up. I was in the pit area hidden from the crowd, where all the competitors' trailers were parked, stretching and gearing up slowly for what I knew was going to be one of the biggest riding challenges of my life. Then Miki came running in, waving everyone toward the track. The X Games officials had to switch the girls' and boys' events due to one of the boys getting injured—which meant we had minutes to get ourselves on the track. I wasn't even in my gear yet! Miki ran through the pits trying to round up all the girls, none of whom were ready. My mom, my dad, and Kicker were hugging and kissing me, trying to say a prayer. I got on my bike and sped toward the gateway that led to the stadium, riding through a dark tunnel into the afternoon sunshine.

I wheeled down a big dirt ramp onto the track, nine other girls alongside me. The stadium was packed—it seemed like more people were watching compared to last year. We had already raced a qualifier to determine our gate picks and the race would unfold like in regular supercross—six laps of sheer, unadulterated gnarliness. My mom told me later that she was so tense, she could barely watch the race. "Tell me when it's done," she said to her friend.

The gate dropped. The ground was exceptionally hard packed and slippery, and because I am so light my tires tend to spin—which is exactly what happened. So I got a horrible start and entered the race eighth out of ten girls. I started pushing forward, slowly but surely, until I made it into second place. The only person in front of me was Jessica.

She had taken a completely different line than the rest of the girls, and it seemed to be working for her—lap after lap, she took the same line, followed the same path, and held on to her lead.

Her consistency, I realized, was where I could attack. I noticed she was jumping the finish-line jump each and every time she hit it, even though it was actually losing her a sliver of time, as the jump was sending her so high in the air. I decided not to take the jump, hoping that staying on the ground would help me gain on her. Slowly, I inched closer and closer to her, until I was right behind her. Then the white flag was waved, indicating the final lap, and I knew I had just seconds to pass Jessica. There was no big maneuver that was going to get me in front of Jessica, just dogged determination—I had to outwit her with my strategy. My determination paid off—she jumped the finish-line jump again and I shaved enough time off to pass her in the whoops in the closing seconds of the sixth lap.

The stadium erupted. The Jumbotron screens started flashing with my name and all around fans were standing up, jumping up and down and clapping. I sped across the finish line in first place, skidded to a halt, and threw my bike down on the dirt. I ran over to the nearest set of bleachers, throwing my goggles and gloves into the crowd. Cameramen and journalists raced over to talk to me, while my mom and dad tried their best to get past the crowds to me. When they did we held one another in the biggest family hug I think we've ever had.

Amid the chaos, the camera flashes, and the swarm of happy faces around me was the perpetual silence in my head, the silence that has allowed me to think clearly in otherwise overwhelming situations. And my thoughts were on all the millions of X Games and action sports who had just seen that nail-biting race on television and who might start asking questions about this funny sport called motocross.

E-Bash came running over; she had won bronze, behind Jessica's silver. Behind her was Lyn-Z, who hugged me in congratulations. I couldn't wait to show her my gold medal too.

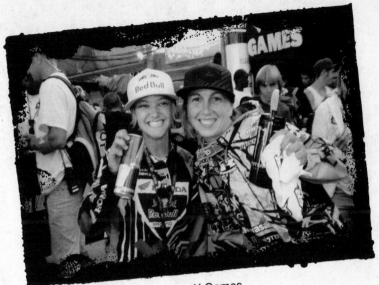

Celebrating with E-Bash at the X Games.

Back at Loretta's . . .

In between races, I visited Loretta's, invited to return as the reigning X Games champion. Loretta's had been such a huge part of my life, and even though I wasn't there to race, it felt like a homecoming of sorts. As always, the atmosphere was carnivalesque. Thousands of racers and their families milled around, eating junk food, playing in the creek, and watching race after race after race. It's always inspiring to me, watching the little kids and seeing how determined they are.

There's a huge billboard at Loretta's that has been there forever, since my dad started racing in 1983, at least. On the billboard are the faces of the top riders, guys like Ricky Carmichael and James Stewart. And this year I saw my face and Jessica's face, up there on the billboard. It was a shock and a huge honor. I hoped all the little girl racers would look up and realize there was a path for them toward the factory teams too, if they wanted it.

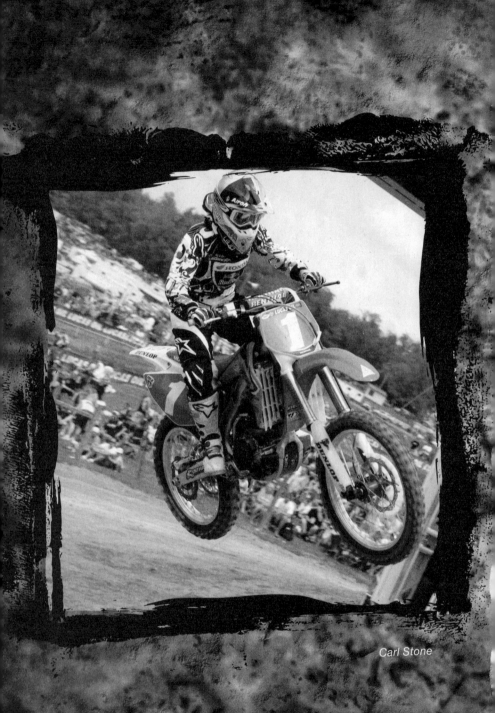

Carl Stone

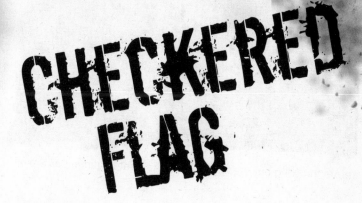

CHECKERED FLAG

Riding with Restraint

At Southwick, Massachusetts, it was pouring rain with temperatures in the low fifties—another mud bath loomed. In theory, I could have locked up the championship by winning at Southwick, but I decided not to race too aggressively, just to be safe. I didn't want to risk my safety in the mud, and Jessica took the race. Nonetheless I still held a forty-one-point lead over her as we headed into the final race of the season. The stage was set for a second championship win for me—provided nothing went wrong at Steel City.

Friday night, before the race on Saturday, I was invited to throw the first pitch out for the Pittsburgh Pirates, which was way cool for a motocrosser. Motocross is the redheaded stepchild of sports, so it was a real honor to be invited to the game.

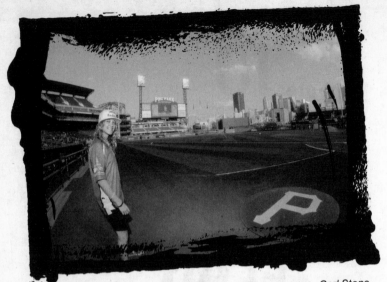

Before throwing out the first pitch at the Pirates game. *Carl Stone*

Holding the ball in my hand on the mound, I felt almost as nervous as I did for a race. My mom translated as the announcer told the crowd a little about me, how I am a member of the Honda Red Bull team and was leading the women in points this season. Then an official gave me the signal, and I threw the ball out as fast and as hard as I could. It traveled eighty feet or so—I've never thought of myself as a pitcher, but apparently they were pretty impressed with my throw.

The next morning, I pulled back the curtains of our hotel room window, feeling a strange sense of déjà vu—this would be the third time I raced Steel City as a pro, and just like last year, predictions of rain had failed to come true. I looked at the beautiful, cloudless September sky. My mom, Kicker, Cody, and I prepared to leave the hotel room and head to the track, and we all knew I was almost certain to take home the champion's trophy, provided I didn't DNF or have some kind of disaster. We had done the math—I only needed to finish in the top eleven in order to be sure of victory. I knew a lot of the top girls would be battling it out for the podium spots, so I kept reminding myself, *Eleventh or better, eleventh or better.* That was all I needed.

On our way to the track my mind kept flashing back to last year—to our post-win celebration food fight at Smokey Bones, people running toward me with bouquets, Jessica giving me her number one plate. Last year the track had worked in my favor; this year, I could only pray for the same kind of luck.

"Hey, snap out of it!" my dad signed a few hours later as he handed me my helmet. We were under the Honda Red Bull Racing rig and I had already warmed up and geared up. My bike looked ready for action. "You ready to win Steel City again?" my dad added, and I smiled.

"OK! Let's do this," I signed, and I motored out of the pit area and over to the starting line for the final race of the 2009 season.

It was pleasantly warm, especially in contrast to the furnace-like conditions we'd endured elsewhere that summer. The unexpectedly clement weather, the almost certain likelihood that I'd win the championship today—was it really going to be this easy? I immediately pushed the thought from my mind. The motocross gods are capricious, and experience had taught me never to take anything for granted in a race. The two-minute board came up and I reminded myself to ride strong and steady and not take any risks. For a rider like me who is used to giving 100 percent, holding back and riding safe took a different kind of skill. Calculated restraint just isn't my MO.

The gate dropped, and it soon became clear that I was the only one riding cautious. The rest of the field was unusually aggressive, and girls were bumping and jostling one another, fighting for points and podium spots.

I saw my friend Sherri Cruse crash hard over a particularly rutted spot in the track—her handlebar ripped a hole through her cheek. Later I would learn she had also fractured her jaw. I tried to stay cool and carried on working my way up through the girls, making it up to second place behind Jessica. *Second isn't at all bad,* I thought as we navigated the track, entering the rutted section once again. Maybe my timing was off because I *wasn't* riding as fast or aggressively as I normally do, but at almost exactly the same spot where Sherri crashed, I lost control, hitting the dirt with a terrible thud. Something cracked and I felt the dull, sickening sensation that all motocross riders know—*something was broken*. Later on I would find out my collarbone had broken clean in two—*snap*.

The bone didn't break through my skin, but it split in two neatly. I had been thrown from the bike but lifted myself out of the dirt and ran back to it, adrenaline surging through my veins. I needed to make a decision—drop out of the race and take care of my broken bone, or carry on and try to save the championship. If I didn't finish in the top eleven, the trophy would go to Jessica. But if I got back on the bike, who knows what kind of a mess my body would be at the end. I looked at my bike—the handlebars and internal cables were completely mangled, but miraculously, the engine was still running. The engine should have cut with that kind of impact. And had it done so, I wouldn't have been able to restart it, because my ignition cables had been so badly damaged. For some reason, the bike had kept running. I took that as a sign from God—I should keep running too. I hauled myself on the bike again and got back in the race.

Although they had no idea I had just broken my collarbone,

my parents could tell something was wrong from the way I was riding. I was wobbling along in seventh place and jumping awkwardly, only stepping things up when a rookie tried to make her way past me. *Good luck, sister,* I thought, flying into a double jump, making sure I could at least stay ahead of her. The pain by this point was still intense, but by the time I dragged myself across the finish line I was running on pure adrenaline. I had come in seventh in the first moto. *I had enough points to win the championship.* Ecstatic as I was, the pain around my shoulders and a new limpness in my arm prevented me from celebrating too hard as I rolled into the pit.

My dad ran over to me. "What's going on?" he signed. I couldn't sign back; it was too painful. He lifted my helmet off my head gently, aware that I was in bad shape.

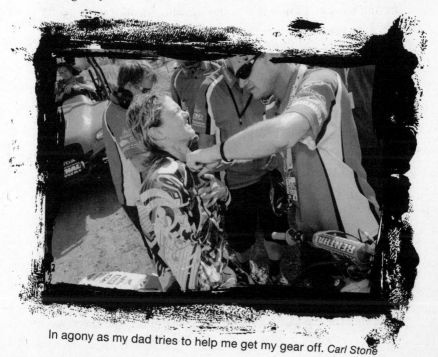

In agony as my dad tries to help me get my gear off. *Carl Stone*

"I think I broke something," I whimpered, gasping for breath.

Up on the podium a huge celebration was under way. I dragged my bruised body up there and tried to smile through the agony. Look at photos and videos from that afternoon and you'll see my grin is a little strained. Someone handed me a number one jersey, which I was supposed to wear on the podium, but I couldn't get it over my head. My right arm was immobilized, hanging down like a chimpanzee's, and I couldn't use it to sign or write autographs because it hurt so bad. It was only when I accepted the trophy with one arm that I allowed myself to break into a real smile. *What a life,* I thought, wishing I had another arm to wave with to the crowd cheering below.

After the race the medical staff gave me a shot and some Vicodin. I went back to watch the rest of the races and started feeling woozy—I knew it was the Vicodin. Most of the time I'll just take the pain rather than the pills—strong in the heart, but weak in the stomach, my mom says. I was shuttled back to the motor home, where I lay down and finally closed my eyes. I was a second-time WMX champion, but there would be no celebratory food fights this year. Tonight, all I wanted was sleep.

Cinderella in a Sling

Post-race X-rays confirmed what we'd feared—it was indeed a broken collarbone. The doctors told me I needed major surgery, in which they would insert a plate and six screws into my body. The prankster in me was looking forward to setting off airport metal detectors for the rest of my days.

But before my surgery, scheduled to take place in Jacksonville, was the big MX Sports dinner celebration, and there was

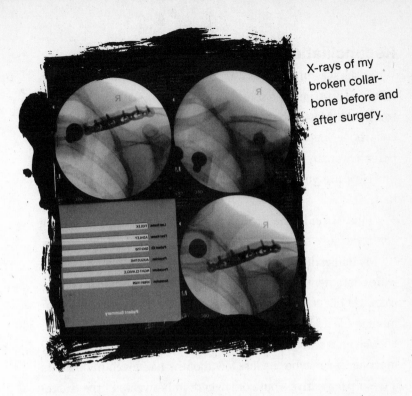

X-rays of my broken collar-bone before and after surgery.

no way I was going to miss that, no matter how beat-up I was. Held at the plush Grand Concourse's ballroom on the riverfront in downtown Pittsburgh, the dinner was for all the top riders, male and female, of the season. Getting dressed for the dinner, I felt like Cinderella . . . Cinderella in a sling, that is. I was too weak to even hold my trophy and was bandaged up. Poor Sherri Cruse was there too and looked even worse than me, what with her broken jaw. I ran into my old friend Ryan Dungey, who had just won the 250 men's championship. He had broken a collarbone once during a race, too. And he seemed impressed that I had gotten back on my bike and finished the race—he hadn't. "You just got back up and rode?" he said, shaking his head. "That's cool." That meant a lot, coming from the men's champion.

Reconciliation

When the season was over we moved out of the house in Canyon Lake and returned to our lives in St. Augustine, which was closer to where the last two rounds of the season were taking place. My collarbone was about to be operated on in Jacksonville, and my parents were by my bedside throughout.

"How are you doing, sweetie?" my mom said, stroking my hair.

"Fine," I said. I had to get good at lip-reading and talking again, because my broken bones were making it painful to sign.

My dad walked into the room behind her holding a Tupperware container that looked like it contained some kind of cheesecake. He put it down by the bed. "For after the surgery—your mom made it," he signed, and kissed my mom on the forehead.

Maybe it's not that easy to walk away from a twenty-year marriage, or maybe the last few months had given my parents a fresh perspective—but somewhere in between all the excitement and broken bones, my mom and dad had decided to give things another shot. They had been going to counseling and had talked through some of the mistakes they had made over the years. Not making time for one another had been a big part of the problem. After my surgery, they had a couple weekend trips planned—down to Epcot Center in Orlando for a food and wine festival, and a trip to Savannah for their twentieth wedding anniversary in November. I was happy for them, especially when my dad moved back into the house.

By October things were almost back to normal again in St. Augustine. Kicker was getting better and better at riding his minibike and we wondered if he too would decide he wanted to race like his big sister—he was getting to that age, after all. And Turbo, one of my bulldogs, seemed to know not to play too rough

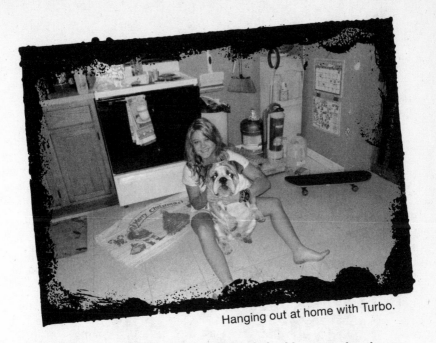

Hanging out at home with Turbo.

with me while I was recovering. Honda had been on the phone to talk about the following year, this book was almost finished, and after so many years focusing entirely on motocross, I was reconnecting with the deaf community again.

Deaf schools were inviting me to visit as a motivational speaker; I was nominated for a Trailblazer of the Year award by Purple Communications, the deaf community's best-known provider of video relay and text relay services; and I was honored at the DEAFestival in Los Angeles, signing autographs and talking to deaf kids about my life in a way I hadn't in a very long time. This time, everyone seemed excited to learn about my life in motocross—even though I hadn't met any of these people before, it felt like I was coming home and catching up with old friends after a long journey.

As usual, though, my injury was preventing me from being as active as I would have liked, and I was having trouble sitting

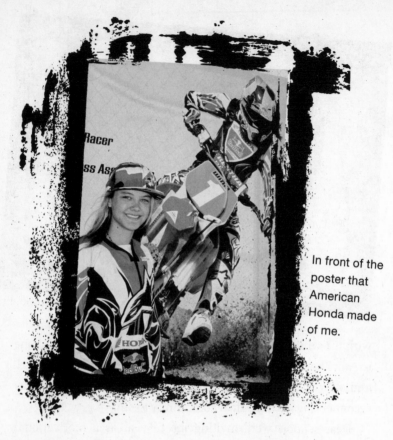

In front of the poster that American Honda made of me.

still for so long—injured or not, there's nothing you can do to stop the motocross itch. And I was thinking about a new coach. We hadn't really figured out whether it should be my dad or not. My dad seemed in no hurry to make a decision. "Let's figure it out later, OK?" he signed, smiling, his gray-blue eyes twinkling the way they always did when he talked motocross. He and my mom had survived one of the biggest tests any family could put themselves through: a life in motocross. It was time for them to put their marriage first. I thanked God for blessing me with such remarkable parents as I hugged my dad.

Next year—on and off the dirt—was going to be a big one.

EPILOGUE: WE'VE ONLY JUST BEGUN

By the end of November of 2009, our postseason relaxation period had drawn to a close and it was time to start gearing up for another year of competition. I had recently turned nineteen and was starting to feel almost like a grown-up, shopping around for houses to buy in St. Augustine, where I would build a track of my own. My mom and dad, it seemed, were continuing to work things out, and Kicker was as sweet and boisterous as ever. I had finally pulled off a backflip on a dirt bike, with Travis Pastrana's help, and the fans were MySpacing and Twittering about it like crazy. Life in the Fiolek household was back to normal—with one exception. Cody had moved back to Wisconsin, leaving so that he could be with his girlfriend. We were still all adjusting to him being gone. He would be hard to replace; not everyone can fit into a family the way Cody had with ours. But we respected his decision. Now we had to start looking around for someone to step into his shoes. It wasn't going to be easy—but then nothing in motocross ever is.

One evening our landline rang, and my dad picked up. He cradled the phone receiver into his shoulder and signed, "It's Keith," meaning Keith Dowdle from Honda. Keith had been a friend and supporter of mine since my amateur years, and we always valued what he had to say. I wondered if Keith was calling to recommend a mechanic as my dad started signing, translating what Keith was saying.

"It's time . . . to think about . . . the future," my dad signed. His face had an intense expression.

My heart dropped and I signed back, "What does he mean, 'the future'?"

"Ashley wants to know what you mean," said my dad, looking as puzzled as I felt. Cody had just left a few weeks ago and we weren't ready for any more big surprises just yet.

"He means . . . another girl," my dad signed. "Honda wants you to help them find the next Honda star. A young amateur girl, like you once were."

My shoulders relaxed and I heaved a sigh of relief. My dad carried on signing: Honda wanted my help in selecting a promising young female racer who would blaze a trail into the pro ranks and follow the example I had set. *What an enormous honor*, not least because 2010 would surely be a crucial year in women's racing. The economy had really taken its toll on motocross, and many pro racers—boys and girls—were facing the prospect of riding the 2010 season with little or no financial backing. If things were bleak in the pro ranks, I can only imagine how the economic downturn would impact amateur racing in 2010.

It felt like only yesterday that I had been making my own transition from amateur to pro—now here I was, aged nineteen, being asked to help usher in the next generation. I thought back to the little girls I had seen hurtling around the track at Loretta's that year, hope and determination in their hearts. I felt excited for them—opportunities lay ahead of them that I had barely dreamed of at their age.

"Tell Keith there are plenty more girls where I came from," I signed to my dad, grinning. *"Tell him we've only just begun."*

ACKNOWLEDGMENTS

I would like to thank the following:

God, for always guiding me and keeping me safe.

My parents, Roni and Jim Fiolek, and my brother, Kicker Fiolek.

American Honda, for having the vision and open-mindedness to support a woman rider in the same way that it supports male riders.

Miki Keller for establishing a women's race series, the Women's Motocross Association, and for always trying to help female riders achieve more.

Caroline Ryder, for making this book happen and for diving headfirst into the crazy world of motocross.

Kirby Kim, my literary agent at William Morris Endeavor.

My editor, Kate Hamill, my production editor, Andrea Molitor, and the whole team at It Books.

All of my sponsors, for believing in me: Red Bull, T-Mobile, Alpinestars, Leatt, Smith Optics, MotoEndurance, Hardcard Motorsport Management, *TransWorld Motocross* magazine, Rockwell watches, and Able Planet.

And my friends and family that have helped me along the way: James Fiolek ("Grandpa Motorcycle"), the Hills, Donn Maeda, Kim Cabe, Rick Wernli, Andrew Campo, and Carl Stone.